THE ACTIVIST
CANCER
PATIENT

THE ACTIVIST CANCER PATIENT

How to Take Charge of Your Treatment

Beverly Zakarian

Foreword by
Ezra M. Greenspan, M.D.
Medical Director
The Chemotherapy Foundation

John Wiley & Sons, Inc.

New York • Chichester • Brisbane • Toronto • Singapore

ISBN 0-471-12026-X

Printed in the United States of America

10 9 8 7 6 5 4 3 2

In my mother's memory

CONTENTS

ACKNOWLEDGMENTS

I've waited years to thank many people:

The generous patients and professionals who shared deeply felt experiences with me so that others might learn. (I've protected their privacy by changing their names.)

"Team Zakarian": Drs. Ezra Greenspan, Carmel J. Cohen, Michael Goldsmith, Larry Norton, Myron E. Schwartz, Kirk Sperber, and Barbara Blum, for their professional skills, personal qualities, and convictions that supported and encouraged this empowered patient. Mike Cohn, my agent, and PJ Dempsey, my editor, for their help, but above all for their belief in me and in this project. What a support group to have!

Jaclyn Silverman and Mary Ellen Siegel, for so much, for so long.

My tennis buddies; Steve; and a few very dear friends who mean so much to me (you know who you are).

The other ten-year survivors of my cancer—my family—for every day together.

FOREWORD

An earlier "don't ask, don't tell" policy hushed the facts of cancer for generations. A tacit conspiracy between doctors, patients, and families allowed the disease to be glossed over, whispered about, closeted.

Today the media and the public talk about cancer constantly and openly, but not necessarily effectively. Cancer patients lack group identity or the social cohesion of the AIDS political forces. Patients' need for active involvement is too often frustrated; they are denied the means of sharing knowledge or of taking their message directly to agencies involved in research and patient care. Federally financed projects, large private foundations, and a growing number of special-interest groups compete to advance their own specific agendas, fragmenting potential power and adding to feelings of helplessness—and dangerous passivity—especially among more informed patients.

In the past four decades, the development of a succession of nearly 200 drugs permitted systemic treatment that is potentially curative in many types of cancer. But who interprets the results of new treatments or determines how and where such treatments should be used for the individual? Clearly, most patients do not actively seek the best treatment and care. Innovative therapy is usually expensive, hard to find, and difficult to have covered by health insurance.

Beverly Zakarian personifies the modern cancer patient—intelligent, informed, and articulate. She has refused to accept cursory advice or feelings of helplessness. She has struggled for, and to some degree achieved, a voice—personal and collective—for the cancer patient in the array of policy-wielding committees, agencies, and boards that make life-and-death decisions on cancer-drug approval and therapeutic availability. As clinical trials test new protocols and medical journals announce breakthroughs, it is insurance-reimbursement policies that increasingly impact the availability of new treatments. Beverly has been a strong leader among cancer patient activists in gaining acceptability for treatment categories such as investigational agents and off-label drugs. We oncologists need this support from our patients; we cannot fight the battle against insurance-industry monoliths alone.

Beverly leads the reader into the dense thicket of political and scientific activities and bureaucratic byways that shape the lives of cancer patients. Her plea is for positive action and for continuous reexamination and investigation of accepted or conventional therapies. Her ten years of personal struggle have taught her to seek out the allies and discern the adversaries and have showed her how to use the system or to circumvent it when necessary. With relentless drive, she has thrust herself into a never-ending battle for empowerment.

I was a lonely pioneer when I began in oncology—the medical possibilities of treating cancer such a revolutionary idea that the field had yet to be named. For fifty years, I've been engaged in the struggle to improve and preserve the lives of my patients through chemotherapy. Now, as these battles continue and other battles emerge to be fought, I am pleased to be part of Beverly Zakarian's crusade, another path to our mutual goal.

EZRA M. GREENSPAN, M.D.
Clinical Professor of Medicine (Oncology), Mount Sinai School of Medicine, New York, and Medical Director, The Chemotherapy Foundation

INTRODUCTION

1985: SHADOWS

I study my naked body in the full-length mirror, frowning. My stomach is definitely bulging. I have a heavy, premenstrual feeling, but my period isn't due yet. I push in on my stomach—it has the resilience of a waterbed—and my waist feels unfamiliar under my hands. Even my clothes fit me like a stranger's: I need large safety pins to close the waistbands of skirts or pants, which leave sculptured red imprints on my fleshy middle.

There's a curious thing about turning points in life. You almost never notice when you're going through one. Only afterward can you look back and say, yes, that was the moment that changed things.

I will always see myself before that mirror, my hands probing my belly, my waist, searching for reassurance. It was evening, the intense light in which I inspected myself flared in the mirror, but behind me there were deep shadows. It was the beginning of everything.

Weeks later, my period arrives, but nothing changes. Perhaps, I reason, it's the early onset of menopause, erratic hormones, water retention. I decide to wait a little longer before going to the doctor again because I'm already being "watched" for changes in what is thought to be an ovarian cyst and fibroids, the dark irregular shadows on hundreds of sonograph pictures that fill my medical file. But I'm afraid to wait too long: In six weeks, my husband and I are joining an educational delegation to China. A cyst can twist or rupture painfully, without warning. I worry that I might find myself in a medical emergency in China, in pain, unable to explain what's happening to me.

The year before, I had reluctantly submitted to a laparoscopy "for

1

my own protection." What was there to be protected against? That fibroids are common in women seemed reassuring at the time; now I'm not so sure. I felt young and invulnerable. Serious things happened to *other* people. Did Dr. N, a GYN surgeon, tell me what he was watching for? He asked about my family history, but it's not one stalked by cancer. There was only my father's sister, skeletal, dying torturously of stomach cancer when I was a child. Indelibly in my memory, she injects herself with painkillers from a syringe thicker than her visible bones because nothing else can be done for her, such was the state of cancer treatment in 1950. And her daughter, my adored cousin Terry, surviving breast cancer after ten years; nothing there to worry about. (For that reason, I will be all the more shaken to suddenly learn that Terry has died of a recurrence of the cancer that no one in our family knew about. My mother calls to tell me this terrible news. At first I don't know who she's talking about. Terry died. "Terry who?" I ask.)

The laparoscopy was not too bad after all. Afterward, a meeting with the surgeon to evaluate the findings: some types of embryonic cells here and there, evidently not a problem because he no longer presses me to have a hysterectomy. At home, Zak queries me anxiously about what the doctor had said. "He said I'm just fine," I shrug.

Then one evening, pain suddenly spirals through my abdomen so sharply that it makes me dizzy, my surroundings for a moment fusing into sparkly white light. The next day, I'm in my doctor's office, prone, exposed. The startled look on her face as she pokes around my reproductive organs frightens me. "The fibroids have grown so much!" she says, with a sudden sharp intake of breath. Dr. M immediately refers me to Dr. B, another surgeon, who sees me the next day. "Hysterectomy," he says. "It all has to come out." He is tall, calm, soft-spoken. It's all perfectly routine. The arrangements are made by his haremlike staff, and I leave with an appointment for surgery.

Two days later, I check into a well-known small hospital where I'm ushered into my sun-filled room as if into an elegant hotel suite, which it resembles. I've bought elegant peach-colored, striped pajamas with a matching robe for the occasion; and I pass the afternoon receiving medical visitors in my best gracious-hostess manner. Some artful flower arrangements arrive from friends, completing the Holiday Hospital effect. This will be a good story to entertain people with later, I think.

Early the next morning, I am prepped and clad in hospital greens so that I feel more like a member of the surgical team than the object of its attention. I bid my husband adieu until we meet again in the recovery room. Several hours later, I drift out of the anesthesia into semiconsciousness to see him standing beside me. He's wringing a handkerchief and frowning. "Hi," I murmur through dry lips.

Abruptly, he breaks into big sobs and blurts out, "You . . . you have cancer."

I open my mouth to respond, but my brain is eradicated by his words and no sound comes out.

Ovarian cancer is hidden, silent. Its symptoms are vague. Like me, most women are not diagnosed until the cancer reaches an advanced stage, when accumulation of fluid (ascites) causes abdominal bloating—and reliance on safety pins hints at a problem. It's lucky for me that I learn about the cancer while still confined to the hospital because I hear only the good news; I can't get out to learn the dismal statistics for ovarian cancer. No one tells me that, of more than 20,000 new cases each year, only one-third survive. My wonderful nurses keep up a stream of encouraging chat about new treatments, about patients who beat it, about how different things are for cancer patients today. By the time I leave the hospital, I'm convinced I'm going to beat cancer, because I'm young and strong and healthy, because this is 1985, and because there are marvelous new treatments.

I wonder if any of them really thought I would make it.

A crisis develops as I make a timetable for going home. My red blood count is very low. I will not be allowed to leave the hospital without a blood transfusion to bring it up to "normal"—hospital regulations. The AIDS virus is already known to have contaminated blood supplies, so I don't want a transfusion—but I fear they could be right. Am I so fragile that a sudden draft could kill me in hours, like a tropical bird I once owned?

One day, unannounced, Dr. M visits me in the hospital, having learned the bad news from the surgeon. Her warm embrace moves me to tears, and I tell her of my blood dilemma. When I reach the part about hospital regulations, the corners of her mouth turn down. "You don't need a transfusion," she says firmly, her Polish accent becoming more pronounced. She explains that, although my count is low, it is not life-threatening and will come up with time and nutrition. This is the reinforcement I needed to give substance to my objection, and I prevail—after I sign a paper that will absolve the hospital of all responsibility for drafts or other bizarre outcomes. It is my first lesson in patient empowerment. It is also the only time a doctor will ever visit me without sending a bill.

Home. The reality of my situation slowly settles around me. I think about the future because I'm scared I won't have one. I also think a lot about the past. How could this have happened?

I telephone Dr. N, the surgeon who was "watching" my condition and who performed the exploratory laparoscopy last year—the one who talked about cell types with me. I take a telephone with a long wire into a small bathroom, close the door, and shut out the light. I want no distractions because I have an urgent question to ask.

When I reach him, I say calmly, "I've been diagnosed with Stage Three ovarian cancer. How can this be? A year ago, you told me that everything was fine."

A pause, then he answers, "Well, no, not exactly."

For a moment, the words don't register, like hearing English spoken with a heavy foreign accent. Not exactly? *Not exactly?* Did that mean that I had ovarian cancer a year ago? A year ago it might not have been Stage Three, advanced, life-threatening. A year!

And then I make a decision: There is no going back to undo the present. I hang up the phone, step out of the bathroom and into my future.

Two weeks postsurgery, I'm to begin chemotherapy at a cancer center near home. I have a slip of paper with the name of an oncologist who is to be my doctor. When I'm ordered to offer myself for an admissions examination, I hop onto the hard, high table, the picture of glowing good health. No one has to tell me because I understand the subtle selection that takes place early in the doctor/patient relationship: Younger, healthier patients are treated more aggressively, which could improve their chances of surviving the disease. Although older patients often have slower-growing or less-invasive cancers than their juniors do, they are less likely to survive, possibly because doctors are unconsciously—or consciously—undertreating them, deciding *for them* that they wouldn't want to go through the rigorous chemotherapy regimen. Not I; I have years of life ahead. I want to be there to see my teenage daughter grow up. I must convince the doctors to invest themselves in my health, my life. I won't be one of the ones who die, I silently promise them, and myself.

My resolve is a very thin whistle in the dark. The first chemotherapy treatment overwhelms my heroics, my will, my control. When the fierce nausea strikes, my body evacuates its contents from every orifice. For hours, I am only semiconscious; finally I sleep, drained of spirit, drained of contents, drained.

Home again. I recuperate, revived by the warm healing spring sunshine that streams through the windows, starting to feel strong, confident, healthy again. Except that my right index finger is paralyzed. I stare at it, will it to bend. It's as if I were trying to move someone else's rigid, accusing digit. And I'm having hearing difficulties. Any sharp sound or loud noise, even speech, rips painfully through me. Everyone around me speaks in low whispers, but I'm worried about what these sudden developments mean. A call to the oncologist is not reassuring. I learn a new word: *neuropathies*. It means a weakness or numbness of the nerves, usually of the extremities (hands and feet)—a toxic side effect of the chemotherapy drugs. He muses, "it's . . . hm, *unusual* . . . to see these effects after the first treatment. They usually develop later." Usually?!!

So that's it, then. My choices are clear. If I continue with the treatment, I might beat the cancer, but I could be paralyzed, handicapped. If I don't, I could die. It seems unreal. I can't picture myself in either scenario. I will have to decide.

A few days later, reading the newspaper over morning coffee, my attention is riveted by a single-column report of a new British drug for treating ovarian cancer. I digest it quickly: The National Cancer Institute is beginning to test carbo-platinum, said to be as effective as the cis-platinum I was treated with, but reputed not to be so poisonous to nerves. It mentions the oncologist in London who developed the new drug, so I call her immediately. Surprisingly, she answers the call, but her frosty tone goes beyond legendary British reserve. I will definitely not be able to secure the drug from her.

She suggests that I enroll in the NCI clinical trial. I make many calls to Bethesda, Maryland, slowly talking my way through the bureaucracy until I reach the right person, meanwhile learning a lot about clinical trials. He tells me that fourteen cancer centers around the country are participating in the carbo-platinum clinical trial; that it's a Phase Three trial, meaning that it will be a long time until results are compiled, but that many patients will be treated with the drug . . . which is all I care about.

Interestingly, I learn that the "new" drug isn't new at all: It's already the leading drug for treating ovarian cancer in Europe and elsewhere. It's new only to us. Instead of approving it for American women on the basis of its proven value in Europe, our Food and Drug Administration (FDA) requires what will turn out to be a total of *ten* additional years of tests. In fact, the new drug has already been in smaller U.S. trials for five years.

Only in 1992 will carbo-platinum finally be proven safe and effective to the FDA's satisfaction. Once approved, it will quickly become a primary therapy for ovarian cancer, because it is equally effective as the earlier form of the same drug, is less toxic, and does not require hospitalization to be administered. While carbo-platinum was going through ten years of *excess* clinical testing, about 200,000 women developed ovarian cancer. Nearly 140,000 women died of their disease, almost all of them burdened by punishing treatment with the only approved drug.

I have a list of the fourteen cancer centers testing carbo-platinum and methodically telephone them all. Fourteen calls later, I understand. I am not going to be accepted on any clinical trial. The single treatment with cis-platinum that I've already had has made me unacceptable to researchers—if I should survive the cancer, they will not be able to prove that only the new drug was responsible. I will ruin the data. And of course the trials are for research, not treatment. They are meant to benefit science, not people with cancer—not until years later, at any rate.

Meanwhile, I've learned about a lot of other things, such as *compassionate release*. It's a loophole through which a patient can get access to a drug that's not FDA-approved when two conditions are met: (1) No other drug is available that can possibly help, and (2) A doctor is willing to do a mountain of paperwork to get it for you. Perhaps I can get carbo-platinum on that basis. All I need is an oncologist who will say that there's nothing else for me. Realizing that it's true stops my heart for a beat. I start shopping for a doctor. And find one.

My friend Lillian, who also has ovarian cancer, recommends her doctor, Dr. G, who has kept her going for several years in spite of Lillian's poor health. I make an appointment and prepare my questions, intending to be businesslike and probing. Instead, when I see him, I am drawn to the intensity of his commitment to saving the lives of people with cancer; to the desk covered with charts that speaks of too many patients; to the feeling that he is really listening to me, hears my concerns. He is exasperated by my tale of the effects of the first chemotherapy, inspects my finger, and remarks wryly that I've been terribly overdosed, probably on a study, which endears him to me (it confirms my suspicions). My agenda not completely forgotten in this strange sizing-up, however, I get answers to my questions. Urgently: carbo-platinum. Can he get it for me? He is impatient, waves off the query. Yes, yes, but what *else* will we do? He will treat me with a combination of four drugs—look at me, I'm young, healthy, strong; I'll be fine. How long a treatment? We'll see.

He suggests we start chemotherapy right away, but I'm afraid. The trip to China is only two weeks off, but he assures me that it will be just a *li-i-i-i-ittle* treatment. I submit, make an appointment. Thumbtacked to the wall above the receptionist's desk is a motto that warns, *Don't Postpone Joy*. Outside the pungent-smelling office, I take deep breaths to cleanse my nose of the metallic, chemical odor. Eventually I realize it has burned its way into memory and cannot be purged.

Traveling in China was unforgettable, the weeks flawed only by the gradual loss of every hair on my head. Engaged in the absorbing struggle for my own life, I find myself deeply identified with the struggle of the Chinese people to lead meaningful and rewarding lives in a tumultuous time, as they move into an unpredictable future.

Our little group rides around in a small comfortable bus, the object of amazed crowds wherever we stop (Western tourists are still a novelty in these pre-joint-venture days). My husband and I become particularly friendly with John, who tells us that he's recently lost his wife to cancer. This trip is a therapeutic change of scenery for him. At first I don't tell him about my own problem, but it must have been visible. I wasn't experienced enough then to recognize the look of cancer.

In memory and in photographs, I see John reaching out to my husband and me, helping us through our own painful time. I stop myself from wondering whether my husband was imagining himself in the future, like John, alone.

We return home to a new priority, chemotherapy. Our lives become organized around my treatment schedule, and Dr. G becomes as much a part of our conversation as any familiar friend. My husband and daughter occupy solar position in our nuclear family, around both of whom I dotingly revolve. Now we change places. Everyone accommodates me. I have a treatment every two or three weeks on Friday morning, so I have the weekend to recover. Each time, I sign a release for the carbo-platinum, swearing that I understand that I'm participating in a research project with a new drug and that I do not expect to benefit from the treatment. Lies, lies. I sign with a clear conscience.

The treatment is a "push"—four different vials of liquid chemicals are plunged into my bloodstream through the prettily named butterfly needle and tubing that dangles from my vein. The chemicals are loathesome, each in its own way, smell, taste, or sensation. After treatment, I go home and immediately go to bed, zonk out with antinausea drugs and sleeping pills. There is always one fitful night spent fighting the queasiness that rises like a knot in my throat as the drugs wear off, waking me punctually every four hours. Some years after this, I will be involved in a struggle to get the FDA to quickly approve a more effective antinausea drug. Patients will tell me that they've gone back to work or out for a meal after chemotherapy, thanks to the new drug. It is an unimaginable improvement.

One day, I have a long, serious discussion with Dr. G about carbo-platinum. I know it is probably responsible for saving my life (so far). Why isn't it available for other women like me who need it? Dr. G explains that the public is only aware of the "consumer watchdog" role of the FDA. But there is a darker side to the protection: The rigid standards that are designed to protect people from exposure to *harmful* drugs are too inflexible for chemotherapy drugs. Although the drugs are toxic, cancer is lethal.

What is the risk of *not* having a drug available to treat a cancer? Too many people die waiting for something that might have saved their lives. It takes approximately ten years and many millions of dollars before a cancer drug is approved for use. Patients always believe that their doctors will be able to get anything possible for them. But they do not understand: The FDA doesn't care whether you or I live or die—there will always be more patients. What's the hurry?

I know what the hurry is for someone with cancer. I leave the doctor's office in a grim mood.

My fifteen-year-old daughter has made herself largely absent since the onset of my illness, going in and out of the house with quick hellos and goodbyes or retreating behind her bedroom door. Those days I'm in bed recovering from treatment, she talks to me from the doorway to my bedroom. I feel sorry for her, having to go through this, and sorry for myself. The idea of leaving her when she might (someday) need me floods me with pain and anxiety and determination to live. I want to be there to see her grow up, but try saying any of this to a fifteen-year-old. I bargain with Fate—please, ten years, please.

One day she brings home an abandoned kitten she has found across the street from our house. It's tiny, sick, barely alive. Its eyes are swollen shut by a festering infection, and it mews pitiably. Although I have misgivings about getting involved in what is clearly going to have an unhappy outcome, my daughter's intensity persuades me. Nothing will do but that we rush the kitten, swaddled in a long-disused doll's blanket, to the veterinarian. He sizes up the situation while he examines the kitten, suggesting gently to my daughter that it is very, very ill. He talks about why it was probably abandoned by its mother, about Nature, and about the possibility of our helping Nature along.

She will have none of it. We must make every heroic attempt. I sense what's really going on here: We're in another life-or-death struggle. I agree to the treatment. The kitten is injected with several medications and, indeed, soon seems to be sleeping more easily, its breathing less labored. We take it home and create a hospital bed in a shoebox, which we place directly under a desk lamp for warmth. My daughter fusses around ward $9^1/_2$B all evening, like an intensive-care nurse.

In the morning, she discovers the kitten has died during the night. She bursts into my room, crying, and comes to my comforting embrace. I hold her around, stroking her hair soothingly. Then, between sobs, she suddenly asks, "Why do things like this have to happen?" Careful, careful, I think; she's not asking about cats. In a few words, I try to explain the inexplicability of life, and I manage to work the unfairness of my own illness into it as an example. She listens, but asks no further questions. After a while, she wipes away her remaining tears and goes to her room to get ready for school. I close the door to my room quietly and go back to bed, where, under the covers, I cry to myself about why things like this have to happen.

During my two years in treatment, and for more years afterward, I have vivid dreams about cancer, dreams of my body as the house in which I live. I dream that I'm with my husband in our house, but there's a terrible problem. On our hands and knees, terrified, we tear away some wooden baseboard molding and peer inside the wall at the wiring and plumbing, branching and snaking every which way. The wiring is glowing red-hot in the dark space. It's on fire! I wake up, my heart racing.

Now that my body's medical treatment is under control and systematic, I'm building up my emotional and spiritual resources. I read *Cancer as a Turning Point*, by Laurence LeShan, and Norman Cousins' *Anatomy of an Illness*. Cousins' hypothesis, that "affirmative emotions [are] a factor in enhancing body chemistry," has become popularized in the notion that, as *Reader's Digest* put it years ago, "laughter is the best medicine." Who knows? So I concentrate on watching comedy movies and videos, and, whenever I laugh out loud, I believe I'm doing myself some good. In fact, I *do* feel better.

I devise an affirmative program for myself. When I'm alone in my car, I roll up the windows and talk to myself out loud (feeling a little silly). "I feel grreeaaaaat!" I'll say, or "I just feel TERRIFIC!!!" It's working—I feel TERRIFIC!!!

Treatment by treatment, a year goes by. My hair is back, I feel great, better than ever. The chemo *must* be working. I supplement my meals with megavitamins. I see a psychologist regularly to deal with my sadness and fears, but also to help me use my strengths. I walk, play tennis, everything. I Don't Postpone Joy.

One day, in the middle of a push, the oncologist shocks me by saying that the next treatment will be my last. I have the option of second-look surgery (still another new term, often called *second-lap look*), another abdominal operation in which the surgeon unzips the hysterectomy incision to look into the pelvis and abdomen to inspect what the chemotherapy has actually done and to biopsy the tissue. I am already monitored by a blood test, CA-125, that measures the level of a substance given off by ovarian cancer cells. My test is nice and low, indicating that the cancer is gone. But how reliable is the test? It's not perfect—it cannot measure a very small amount of cancer, but a very small amount can quickly grow into measurable tumor. Ovarian cancer is a disease with a high probability of recurrence. Every indication is that I'm cancer-free, but is it safe to stop chemo?

I'm not sure what to ask, because it seems so sensible. If I've been lucky enough to have cancer in a site that *can* be directly examined by an experienced surgeon, why not? Going through another abdominal operation is not a picnic, but it could reassure me that I've been cured. It's reassurance I want, and I agree to it.

They find microscopic cancer cells. I need more chemotherapy.

1986: LIGHT

I'm distraught, depressed. I was so *sure*. How could I feel so well and still have cancer? The (new) surgeon comforts me. It's not all bad news—the small tumor "seedlings" that were left after the original surgery are gone, killed by the chemotherapy. "Look at it this way," he urges. "The treatment worked. You just need more." I try, but I understand better than before what a persistent and wily enemy is cancer.

Another year of chemotherapy, the treatments spaced slightly farther apart. I can handle them a little better now, too, finally having found the combination of antinausea drugs and sleeping pills that works best. I am encouraged when tingling feelings in my paralyzed finger give rise to slight tremors of movement that gradually restore it to normal functioning. I demonstrate bending my finger to everyone as if it were a miracle—it is to me. My hearing problem also was gradually disappearing.

I try to get on with my life. I start a graphic design studio with a friend. We have an exciting and promising year, but a collapsing economy takes out our biggest client and then us. I ponder what to do with my suddenly more-precious life.

My friend Lillian is dead. She leaves money in her will for a memorial coffee klatch for a group of close women friends. When we have the gathering we reminisce about the ways Lillian's life touched ours. Others' memories are mostly funny or happy, but mine are about sickness and hospitals. Cancer was our bond. The afternoon leaves me depressed. If Dr. G couldn't save her, how can he save me? Can anyone be saved? This line of thinking shocks me into an accounting: *Everyone I knew with cancer is dead.* I don't know anyone with cancer who is alive. I feel a cold squeeze of fear in my stomach.

Someone suggests I join a cancer survivors' group run by a social service organization. I'm not entirely finished with treatment—not quite ready to begin "surviving." The social worker who interviews me is sympathetic to my situation. She places me in a group where I finally meet people who have had cancer *and are still alive.* There is a man who'd had a massive brain tumor ten years before; two women recently out of treatment for colon; two women with breast, me with ovarian—what a lot of diseased body parts we represent. I'm teary and emotional, encouraged by their stories, but at the same time dismayed: I find out that survivors face a different set of problems, different issues. I've been so preoccupied with getting rid of the damned disease that I didn't even think about the fear of it *coming back.*

The second year of chemotherapy ends. Once more I am in the hospital, hopeful that this time will prove the demon disease has been exorcised by the powerful magic of chemotherapy. I don't sleep well the night before the surgery. At dawn, I'm restless and ready for the gurney that arrives to take me to the operating floor. I study the ceilings of the corridors through which I'm wheeled. Last time I went this route, I was lighthearted, full of anticipation that the procedure would confirm that I'd put an end to cancer. Now, my heart is heavier. I know the possibilities—and I fear the *im*possibilities.

The glistening green operating room to which I'm delivered bustles with green-capped, -gowned, -bootied people. A few cross-checks confirm that the right patient has been transported and that I know what I'm there for. The surgeon greets me, then quickly the green dissolves into blackness.

I wake up, wide awake, in the now-familiar, blindingly white recovery room. I'm desperate to know the results, but it will be about five days before all of them are ready. Over the next few days, news from pathology trickles in. The frozen sections: NED (No Evidence of Disease). Forty-seven biopsies: NED. And the pelvic washings that contained residual cancer last time? We wait.

One quiet afternoon, a friend is visiting when the phone rings. The instant I recognize the voice of the surgeon, I close my eyes tightly, then cover them with my hand, a double withdrawal into darkness and isolation—the same way I had closed the door and turned out the light to speak with another surgeon two very long years ago. My only reality is his voice in my ear: "The washings are back," he says. "They're clean."

"Clean." I repeat his word, my voice wavering. I thank him for calling and hang up the phone, all without removing my other hand from my shut eyes. Some time passes before I am able to come out of the darkness, into light and life.

1987—AND AFTER

One autumn evening, preparing to go to bed, I glance at myself passing the mirror. Something about the angle and the light stops me—I've seen many selves reflected in this panel in this same way. The images meld. I tighten the sash of my bathrobe briskly and start to move away when I'm suddenly overwhelmed: The pajamas I'm wearing, the robe, they're my hospital clothes! I bought them specifically to take to the hospital a lifetime ago, when all this started. An odor seems to cling to them: the sharp smell of chemicals, the stink of hospitals, the smell of cancer! It gets stronger; fills my nose and throat—*suffocating* me.

I tear them off, leaving them in a heap on the floor. They've been washed too many times for them to smell of anything. I'm imagining it. I gather the pieces up, throw them into the wastebasket, thinking, Get OUT of my life! Suddenly I'm aware that these garments have been part of my journey through hell. I can't throw them away like meaningless garbage. You don't just throw away a worn-out American flag, do you? It's dispatched ritually, burnt with ceremony.

A few weeks later, I have a pajama-burning party, surrounded by the good friends who helped me be a normal person in abnormal times. A galvanized-steel garbage can on my terrace serves as pyre to the sacrificial garments. They burn quickly in a hot bright flame. The season's first soft snowfall has begun and it's cold outside, so we watch from indoors. The room lights are out, but the blaze illuminates our somber faces, the heat radiating through the glass. We share the quiet minutes in which I am cremating the past, cremating cancer. I do not try to hide my tears.

But if you're like me, when you're done with cancer, you're never sure it's done with you. That twisting spasm, that sharp stabbing pain, what was that? With periodic batteries of tests, you prove over and over again to yourself (and your doctor) that you're okay, and you learn to deal with your own anxiety.

When I go for checkups, though, we talk about the problems of people with cancer. I'm indignant. My life has been threatened! But for the cancer establishment, I'm business as usual. If I hadn't found the best new treatment for myself and a doctor who treated me as more than an object on an assembly line, I wouldn't be here. I'm angry that there isn't more information available, angry at the way people like me with cancer must fend for themselves. I passionately want to *do* something. But what?

Dr. G invites me to a meeting at which he discusses cancer-patient issues. He offers a doctor's perspective, explaining how federal restrictions on drug approvals frequently prevent him from treating patients with the most effective combination of drugs. This strikes a sensitive nerve in some of the others present who, like me, have experienced difficulty in gaining access to new medicines. We share the view that access to treatment is the most important problem for patients and that it's a patients' rights problem. We agree to work together: Since there is no cancer activist organization, we'll become it.

We designate ourselves CAN ACT, the Cancer Patients Action Alliance. It has a firm, determined sound. I design letterhead and, in January 1990, we're in business. We decide after some debate not to waste time forming another free-standing organization with members, contributions, annual meetings, and such, but to educate and form coalitions with existing cancer organizations around our issues. We expect cancer patients to work in their own interests when we show them what they are; so we plan CAN ACT to be a volunteer organization. I am, surprisingly, elected president.

We survey patient organizations and learn that they are virtually entirely *care*-based: providing advice, social services, psychological counseling, occasionally financial or transportation services. What about patients' rights to treatment? What about patient representation at the National Cancer Institute? What about the escalating health insurance problems facing people with cancer? No groups are active in these areas. We have our agenda.

It was the beginning of medical advocacy, and anything seemed possible. AIDS activists had already marched across America, across Washington, and across the roof of the FDA. Their "in your face" tactics had been rewarded by victories against powerful federal regulatory authorities, and we only wanted for cancer what they got for

AIDS: more sensible, flexible regulatory policies that would get more drugs to more people more quickly, to help them fight for their lives.

One of CAN ACT's founding Board members learns in 1992 that the FDA has a small, little-known office with big-time power. The Office of AIDS Coordination, established within the FDA (and, revealingly, reporting directly to the commissioner) to mollify the AIDS patient community, has powers broad enough to coordinate *all* government agencies to stimulate the rapid development and approval of new treatments for AIDS and its related conditions.

We think, what about cancer? I've drafted lengthy position papers justifying the need for equal cancer-patient representation at the agency—nicely reasoned, measured, polite statements. Never having heard of our fledgling group, though, FDA files our letters away without feeling obliged to respond. Mystified—and miffed—after months of one-way communication, I finally telephone, realizing that activists don't write polite letters! I am passed from voice to voice until I reach a woman who has cancer in her family, knows the issues, and takes an interest in CAN ACT. She finds the letters, and sees that they land on the right desk. We get a meeting with the Commissioner, the very first time that cancer patients have done so. We take pictures of it, like tourists.

Having entree at the agency, a bargaining chip, we manage to form an ad hoc coalition with a few other cancer organizations about FDA issues, and a historic first meeting of grassroots cancer-patient organizations is the gratifying result. Two more years of work results in an expansion of the AIDS office to encompass cancer and other life-threatening diseases. We don't have the clout of AIDS, and never will, it seems. But CAN ACT has made a real contribution to the advancement of patient interests.

The coalition of patient organizations quickly fragments, dissipating the force that might have come from our joint representation of millions of people. It's not comforting to be assured by many people that anyone involved in grassroots organizing has had a depressingly similar experience.

Nonetheless, CAN ACT opens my life to unexpected possibilities. I write, speak, and travel, meeting thousands of patients who are frustrated with the way things are, hope for change, yet are not "activated" to work in their own interests. It's hard for people going through treatment to be activists, but they drift away from the commitment afterward, it appears. People want simple answers, and they want someone else to do the work. It won't work that way.

I start *bulletin*, the organization's newsletter, and *Cancer Frontline*, a slender blue publication that presents selected clinical trials in plain, nonmedical English (a unique educational service). *Frontline* is very well received by patients and medical professionals alike when we mail it out, and, for many months afterward, we get calls from social work departments in hospitals requesting additional copies. But an organization cannot run on individual contributions, we learn, so we try to develop contacts with drug companies, the deep pockets in cancer.

We reason that we have critical interests in common: We want more drugs to treat cancer and we want them developed and approved more quickly. But our approaches for support are responded to tepidly. It finally dawns on us that they are in an ambiguous situation: FDA approval of a drug can be worth millions or more to a company. Having skillfully engineered a working relationship with the agency that polices and regulates them, they will not risk their vast profits and laboriously nurtured connections by becoming associated with CAN ACT, an organization *confronting* the FDA!

We squeak out another issue of *Cancer Frontline* with minimal pharmaceutical funding, but we cannot even thank the contributors by name, at the firm request of their lawyers. Another company dangles the offer of sustained funding of the publication as a patient-education project, then rejects us in favor of a feel-good exhibition. Discouraged, I fold the publication. For the next two years, people continue to call and request copies, adding to my dejection.

But the intense immersion in policy issues is also satisfying. For five years, I travel regularly to FDA meetings to protest the lack of patient involvement in hearings that recommend (or reject) new drugs, the lone representative of patient interests present. The regulations mandate consumer representation, but they are flouted in both letter and spirit by a cynical bureaucracy, that *appoints* supposed "consumer representatives" from a slate of "authorized" groups. Several "consumers" have been physicians, not your typical cancer patient. At meetings of oncology advisory committees, I am asked to limit my remarks to five minutes or so (after traveling more than three hours), because there is important business to transact.

Although the attitude toward patient representation at the FDA changes slowly for the better, we are still marginalized—never seated to represent our own interests on panels nor able to participate in decisions that could have dramatic effect on people with cancer. Why? Because they know there will be no outcry from patients, no matter how flagrant the abuse of power.

CAN ACT participates in founding what becomes the National Breast Cancer Coalition, which succeeds in raising the public profile of cancer—but *only* of breast cancer. Once more, the cancer community has succeeded in splintering itself, fragmenting its power and potential.

The accomplishments of cancer advocacy in the past half-decade have opened a new chapter in the fight to conquer cancer, for individual access to treatment, and for advances against the disease. For the first time, energy and momentum for change coming from the public has filtered up to the professionals.

But we need more voices. Where are the patients? Where are *you*? Ten million people who have had cancer should have the collective clout of the largest interest group in the country. Instead, our voice in Congress is a mere whisper. We will remain health's silent compliant majority until everyone understands that we are members of the same enormous interest group.

If a million people like you each year became advocates for the best treatment for yourselves and stayed as hands-on activists for cancer afterward, think how we could change things for ourselves and those we love.

1

WHY BE AN ACTIVIST PATIENT?

There is no such thing as "a touch of cancer." Cancer is almost always life-threatening. If you have even the most innocuous-seeming cancer, you should be treated as if your life depended on it. It might: Any cancer can kill.

Cancer is a *type* of disease, not just one disease. There's my cancer and yours—forty-six common types of cancer, several hundred different cancers in all. *Your* cancer is as unique as you are. The treatment you receive must be targeted to your own disease.

FINDING THE BEST TREATMENT OPTIONS

Because cancer is not one disease, no single treatment is universally effective. Because it is not like other diseases, treatments known to be effective for one type of cancer may prove useless for another. As a result, cancer treatment has become something of a "cottage industry" in which responsible oncologists may hold diverse, often conflicting, views about the appropriate course of treatment for an individual.

Your first course of treatment is your best hope, so you must become expert in your own case to be sure of getting the best possible treatment for yourself. No one has more to gain. No one cares more about the outcome.

PATIENT EMPOWERMENT: ADVOCACY TO ACTIVISM

Too much about cancer debilitates and depresses cancer patients. All of us have strengths, but we don't call upon them much, except to manage the emotional impact of the diagnosis and treatment. When we have no sense of control over events, naturally we have greater fear about what will happen to us. Being *empowered* permits us to participate in our own important decisions with a *sense* of control, as well as actual control. It can be therapeutic.

Empowerment gives us the right to assume responsibilities for things that concern us. It enables us to act in our own interests, whether we are *talking* about cancer or *doing* something about it.

Just as people with cancer have not felt they had the power to do much to help themselves individually, most of us with the disease have not recognized that we are people with important interests in common. Cancer as a public issue is awakening from its long sleep because:

- *There is more than one choice of treatment for many forms of cancer.* Patients are becoming educated to the importance of their involvement in the decision-making process because there is often no clear "best way" to treat someone's disease. Everyone wants to be sure of getting the best possible treatment.
- *Delivery of health care services is changing.* The public is losing control over choice of doctors and treatments at the same time that it is becoming aware of the need to have that flexibility. Nowhere is this more true than with cancer, and doctors and patients alike are concerned about the impact of health care reform.
- *Medical advocacy is an idea whose time has come.* A decade of forceful AIDS activism energized treatment activists in many other diseases who recognized that health has become politicized. Attention, funding, and progress have gone to the diseases that become influential.
- *The nature of cancer advocacy has changed.* Until now, advances in cancer treatment have been driven by health or social work professionals seeking funds to discover the cure. For the first time, grassroots cancer organizations, with a larger agenda, are demanding a voice in setting cancer policy and priorities.

When you finish reading this book, you will have an education in why you must understand how your own cancer is different from anyone else's, in the strategies necessary to get the information you need to become your own expert, and, finally, in how you can turn your personal advocacy into activism—and why you must.

CANCER TREATMENTS: WHY ARE THERE SO MANY?

People Are Different

Why should patients have to fight for their own lives when they are paying highly skilled people very well to do just that for them? Simply put, *cancer is different in different people, in critically important ways.*

It all begins with you. People differ in biochemical and psychological makeup in as many subtle ways as they differ in appearance, although all have the recognizable elements of humanity. Because of differences among us, and in the nature of cancer and cancer treatments, no doctor can guarantee that any one treatment will work for you or me.

There is not one cancer that *someone* hasn't survived, no matter how deplorable the statistics. So, you may as well hope and plan to be the one in a million, or in ten, or in two, because neither you nor your doctor knows how it will all work out. That hope and those plans should be dynamic. Too much reliable evidence has accrued demonstrating that active involvement in your own treatment has beneficial effects. (See Chapter 8.)

As research progressively closes in on the infinitesimally small basis of the ways in which people differ from one another while seeming so much the same, diagnosis and treatment inevitably will evolve. Even now, about fifteen cosmic minutes after the dawn of understanding of some of the causes of cancer, medicine is fractured by controversy. Does the presence of an *oncogene*, a gene for cancer, mean that a person will inevitably develop cancer? It does not. Does the absence of a hereditary gene for a familial type of cancer mean that you are in the clear? It doesn't mean anything of the sort. One of the very few things known with certainty about ovarian cancer is that it is uncertain: Even in families with one of the known hereditary forms, any one woman may never develop the disease—or she may develop a nonhereditary type, unrelated to her apparent genetic destiny. (And therein lies the whole troubling issue of genetic testing.)

Understanding how cancer can be prevented from developing is an urgent question. Until it can be answered, medical research is concentrating on finding ways to maximize the effect of treatment by tailoring it to the individual cancer.

Cancers Are Different

Cancer is a catchall name for a complex of two hundred or more different diseases that have in common primarily the characteristic of uncontrolled cell growth. The breathtaking diversity of life—plant or animal—is based on variations of the common building block, the cell. Normally, refined and delicate genetic-control systems permit cells to grow by division of preexisting cells; to differentiate (become specialized) in order to perform different functions, such as becoming brain or red blood cells, and, finally, to die when the cell's product or its participation is no longer needed, when fresh, newly differentiated replacement cells can maintain healthy functioning.

When something damages these complex controls and cell division cannot be stopped, cells replicate ceaselessly, piling up and leading to the formation of tumors. Tumor cells live longer because they lose the ability to respond to the normal controls that make them die. To make matters worse, tumor cells acquire some additional undesirable characteristics, such as invasiveness, and they are able to disguise their malignant character from the immune cells that recognize and attack cellular invaders.

Many factors are known to originate or stimulate the development of cancer, but it is not yet known what makes certain cancers happen to certain people. Cancer is a *heterogeneous* disease, meaning that it is very individualized (the opposite of *homogeneous*, meaning all the same). The same cancers in different people may respond to treatment in unpredictable ways; and in each individual, the cancer may change over time. Tumors can become resistant to drugs that were formerly effective in controlling them, so it is important that a range of therapies be available.

Oncology is an art because the course of each patient's treatment is not secure. Science is based on repeatable, demonstrable, predictable results. If treating cancer were as "scientific" as, for example, setting a broken bone, it would be better for cancer patients. But it is not; it is more trial and error.

"Cancer chemotherapy is often more empirical than rational," say the authors of *The Anticancer Drugs*. "[It is] a fact that does not detract from the intelligence or dedication of the clinicians and scientists involved; rather, it speaks to the complexity of the issues they face."*

Understanding is basic to empowerment. Understanding how cancers differ, you'll know why you—and only you—must become the expert in your own case. Understanding how treatments differ, you'll know why you must become an informed medical consumer. Understanding what is happening will make you feel more confident of your own ability to participate responsibly, secure in the expertise of your professional team.

Don't be too hard on yourself if you cannot understand everything at once: Learning is a process.

THE MANY TYPES OF CANCER

Similar types of cancers develop from similar tissue, regardless of where in the body they occur.   The same few types of cells, performing the same functions, can give rise to the same type of tumors in different organs. Cancers are classified according to the type of cell they contain:

*   *Carcinomas.*   These are solid tumors of epithelial tissue— tissue that covers surfaces in the body, such as the layers of skin, and that lines hollow internal organs, such as the stomach and the uterus. Because epithelial tissue may consist of several cell types in single sheets or layers, an organ may have more than one kind of carcinoma.
*   *Adenocarcinomas.*   These are solid tumors of epithelial tissue that is structured into glands, which are like little bags that generate specialized fluids. Some glands "leak" the substances, such as hormones, into the blood circulation (like oil through a paper bag).

*William B. Pratt, et al.; *The Anticancer Drugs*, 2nd ed. (New York: Oxford University Press, 1994), 15.

Others pour the fluids, such as sweat, into channels that carry them to specific locations.

Lymphomas. These are most often solid tumors of the lymph nodes. Lymph nodes are special small glands that dot the lymphatic system, a network of vessels that transports lymph to all parts of the body and interacts closely with the blood circulatory system. Lymph is the fluid that contains the specialized cells of our immune systems, primarily the disease-fighting T cells and B cells. However, when those cells become malignant, the disease is a leukemia.

Leukemias. These are cancers of several types of blood cells. All blood cancers are diffuse and do not form solid tumors. Blood cells develop within bone marrow, which lies in cavities in the spongy center of bones. Most leukemias involve abnormal T or B white cells, but occasional malignancies are found in red blood cells, which transport oxygen, and in platelets, the small cells that clot to stop bleeding at the surface of wounds.

Sarcomas. These are solid tumors of the tissue that structures, supports, and connects organs. The skeleton, muscle, cartilage, ligaments, and fat are all connective tissue, and so are vessels of the blood and lymphatic circulatory systems. There are many distinct types of sarcoma; it can arise from the bone marrow, even from one or another area of a specific bone, or from the different soft tissues, depending on the type of cells in which it started.

Tumors can be solid or dispersed in fluid. Bone, brain, lung, and most other types of cancer develop as solid tumors, while leukemias (cancers of cells in the blood) do not form solid tumors. The cancerous cells circulate, diffused, in the bloodstream. Many cancers spread by means of a circulatory system, but that is a metastasis, not a primary tumor.

Different organs produce different tumors. Solid tumors arising in organs such as the liver, lung, or uterus are separate, distinguishable cancers and respond to different treatments. Cancer arising in an organ can be identified as that type, different from cancers of other organs, even adjacent ones. For example, although there are several types of ovarian cancer, all of them are identifiably ovarian, and not cervical or uterine or any other female reproductive organ. (See *metastasize*, p. 25.)

One type of cancer in an organ may have different forms. Cancer of one type may have subtypes, depending on the tissue or cell type from which it developed. Skin, for example, has several layers of cells of different types, each of which can form cancers with different properties:

- *Basal cell carcinoma*, the most commonly occurring, generally least-dangerous skin cancer, originates in the deepest layer of epidermal cells, although it appears on the surface of the skin.
- *Squamous cell carcinoma*, the second most common form of skin cancer, arises from keratinocytes, cells that make up the protective outside layer of the epidermis. It may develop relatively harmlessly toward the skin surface, or it can infiltrate more deeply and dangerously into the lower dermis.
- *Melanoma* is the cancer of special pigment-producing cells called melanocytes, which are found in the skin, eyes, and elsewhere. It is the most malignant of all cancers. To complicate the picture, melanoma itself has subclassifications based on variations of the cell shape.

Different cell types may be found within one tumor. It may be that tumors start with one aberrant cell that reproduces (clones) itself again and again to form a cluster that grows into a tumor (the "clonal" theory). Or perhaps they develop from many cells in the same region that have been damaged by exposure to a carcinogenic insult like an X ray (the "field" theory). How tumors begin is not yet really understood. Nonetheless, it is known that, as tumors grow, different clusters of cells develop, some of them becoming resistant to drugs and others remaining sensitive to one or more drugs. By the time a tumor is large enough to be clinically detectable, it contains a mixed population of drug-resistant and drug-sensitive cells. Drug resistance is increasingly recognized as an important cause of treatment failure, so more attention is being directed by scientists to outwitting the devious mechanisms that permit cells to render lethal chemicals harmless.

Primary, metastasized, and recurrent tumors differ. The primary tumor is the one in the original site (*in situ*). If cells from the primary tumor *metastasize*, that is, either spread to another location on an adjacent organ or travel in blood or lymphatic circulation to more distant sites, the new tumors that form are the original (primary) type. Breast cancer, for example, frequently metastasizes to bones or lungs, but the tumor that forms there is still a breast cancer. A small percentage of metastatic cancers cannot be precisely identified as to their origin and are known as cancers "of unknown primary site."

Recurrent tumors or metastases are not exactly the same as the original tumor. Cancer cells may become genetically unstable and develop resistance to treatment drugs, so a new combination of drugs or a different mode of therapy is usually necessary for treatment to be effective.

Some cancers are related. A great deal of research at present is focusing on genetic or hereditary factors in hope of understanding what makes some people more likely to develop cancer. Familial links might mean inheriting not only the same type of cancer, but one of several related cancers. For example, families with a specific inherited syndrome show higher-than-expected incidence of breast cancer in women, more prostate cancer in men, and more colon cancer in both sexes.

CLASSIFYING TUMORS

There are several ways to classify the size and extent of tumors. Biopsy or surgical removal of a tumor permits it to be studied for specific details so that treatment decisions can be carefully tailored to your particular cancer.

•   *Staging* is a measure of tumor size and the extent of spread, if any, beyond the primary site. It describes the stage the cancer had reached *when it was discovered.*

In principle, the numerical staging of different types of cancer infers the same thing.

Stage 1 denotes any localized tumor.
Stage 2 describes a tumor still restricted to a region, perhaps with nearby lymph node involvement.
Stage 3 indicates the presence of distant metastases.

Staging of some types of cancer is further defined by alphabetical additions, as Stage 1A or Stage 3C.

Because the organs surrounding the primary site are different and the way tumors spread may differ, the description is not exactly comparable from type to type or case to case. To add to the confusion, each type of cancer may have more than one standard system for measuring and describing the tumor. Non-Hodgkin's lymphoma, for example, may be classified by the Rappaport Classification, by the Lukes and Collins system, or by the prevalent standard description known as the Working Formulation.

In a much-needed attempt to standardize the description of the extent of a cancer, a new staging system called TNM is being instituted:

T stands for *tumor* and is accompanied by a number from 0 to 4, indicating increasing tumor size.

N stands for degree of spread to the lymph *nodes*. The accompanying numbers 0 to 4 indicate increasing distance outward from the tumor.

M stands for the presence of *metastasis*. The accompanying numbers 0 or 1 indicate the absence or presence of metastasis.

Although the TNM system seems logical, in fact it is complicated by the very complexity of cancer and may be inadequate by itself to provide more information than the staging numbers 1, 2, and 3. At any rate, if you hear it discussed or see it on your reports, you will know what it's about.

Tumor grade is a classification of tumors based on study of the individual cells that make up the tumor. Tumors are classified as *high-grade* or *low-grade*—a designation that is confusingly based on an *inverse* description of the component cells' ability to differentiate—perform their biological function. High-grade tumors have a high cell turnover rate—the cells divide more frequently, they are faster-growing, fewer of the cells differentiate, and they may be more aggressive. Low-grade tumors have a lower cell turnover rate—the cells are more differentiated, they grow more slowly, and they are less aggressive and invasive.

- *Lymph node status* measures extent of the disease by indicating how many lymph nodes have become involved. Greater distance from the site of the original tumor implies more spread.

 • *Hormone receptor status* describes the likelihood that breast cancer has been stimulated to grow by either of the prevalent female reproductive hormones, estrogen or progesterone. Thus, it can also be used to predict whether a tumor is likely to respond to hormonal therapy. Because both male and female reproductive systems are modulated by hormones, tumors that develop in them are also affected by hormones. Hormone antagonists, which are substances that prevent hormones from exerting their energizing effect on tumor growth, can be used as treatments.

THE DIFFERENT GOALS OF TREATMENT

You and I may have goals for treatment that differ from the goals of researchers and even from some of our doctors. Scientists have "clinical endpoints" whose standards for determining effectiveness may be too narrow to be meaningful to us. (See Chapter 5 for fuller discussion of ethical issues in clinical research.) As a result, there is a lively controversy about the value of treatments that cannot cure but might prolong survival.

For us, cure is certainly preferable, but disease-free survival, longer disease-free intervals, and other less-absolute measures of survival are acceptable goals of treatment. If you are to understand how decisions are made about which drugs are effective and which drugs you can be treated with, you should know what the professionals think are realistic options:

Cure

The medical standard for *cure*—a word to use cautiously—varies with the type of cancer. To most people, a cure is simply cancer that never recurs. To scientists, a cure is effected when the death rate of cancer survivors is *statistically* the same as that of the general population, meaning that people are no longer dying *from the cancer.* For a few types of cancer, that might be in approximately five years; but for others, notably breast cancer, a *survival plateau*—when people are not dying of the disease—cannot be safely established for ten or more years. And those are years of *disease-free survival*, which is different from *survival*.

Disease-Free Survival

People with the best chance of *long-term survival,* or cure, are those who *never* have a recurrence—they have infinitely long disease-free survival. Any recurrences diminish the probability of long-term survival, and each recurrence increases the possibility that there will be others. For most cancers, the risk of relapse is greatest soon after (apparently) effective treatment but diminishes with the passage of time.

Disease-Free Interval

This is the period of time between active episodes of disease. It is significant because shorter intervals may mean that resistances are developing, which can have treatment implications. In any case, the variety and inventiveness of modern treatment contributes to the probability that more patients will live longer than was formerly possible. In that regard, cancer is considered a *chronic* disease, with acute phases in treatment alternating with dormant phases (remission).

Survival Value

If a drug cannot cure a cancer (bring about a permanent disease-free condition), perhaps it can delay the onset of recurrence or metastasis. Although someone might eventually die of the disease, it would be of disease that recurred *later* than expected. The drug would be said to have *no survival value* if the treated patient did not live any longer than someone who was not treated with the drug. Nevertheless, someone who has had a longer disease-free interval has arguably had a better quality of life, although medically the endpoint has not changed.

Reasonable Expectations

Try to define reasonable expectations for your own treatment goals with your doctor. It is not wise to do it too early in your treatment when not enough information may be available. Some cancers are curable, but many more are treatable.

THE FIVE-YEAR SURVIVAL QUESTION

Medical textbooks, even those from as recently as the early nineteenth century, show horrific and disfiguring cancers afflicting all body parts: facial features, limbs, genitalia. These disquieting pictures indicate that cancers progressed to very advanced stages over several years because diagnosis was impossible until the disease became growths or swellings that festered visibly or interfered with normal functioning.

Five-Year Figure

If patients weren't killed by the primitive medical treatment available and didn't succumb to the disease or the host of infections that commonly invaded, they were likely to survive. People who were alive five years afterward were considered cured. Five years became fixed in the popular consciousness as the standard, a marker for cure that continues to our time.

How valid is it today? The idea of *cure* lingers from that simple understanding of the nature of cancer. From that point of view, almost half of all cancers diagnosed today are cured (if only for five years), which conflicts with any commonsense understanding of the meaning of the word *cure*.

At the time that five years acquired mythic significance, nothing was known about secondary cancers, nor about the phenomenon of late-developing cancers that result from treatment (there *was* no effective treatment). So it is not a question of surviving five years, and then walking away, relieved that it's over and done with. The real difficulty is learning to live with uncertainty.

Does Earlier Detection Mean Longer Survival?

The technology of diagnosis enables many cancers to be detected well before they are very noticeable or interfere with vital functions. Earlier diagnosis usually leads to earlier treatment, which may mean a better prognosis.

Yet earlier detection may be immaterial to the question of five-year survival. There are scientists who believe that although cancers may be *detected* earlier, patients will not live any longer with treatment than they would have if the cancers were detected later. And they argue that broad-scale screening procedures to detect cancers in the general population are not effective, so they are not cost-effective for society.

Follow-up diagnostic tests for recurrent cancers are dogged by the same controversies. Is a woman with breast cancer better off knowing *sooner* that her cancer has recurred if medicine cannot offer more or better treatment? There is little unanimity among physicians about the value of early detection, but we patients are understandably less objective about the issue and tend to want all possible measures taken.

THE AFTEREFFECTS OF TREATMENT

When few people survived cancer for five years, there was not much opportunity to understand its aftermath. Thanks to modern techniques, many people live more than five years, their cancers either cured or controlled. But follow-up studies of long-term survivors have shown that there is a surprising downside: The chance of recurrence or of the development of an entirely new cancer is made much greater by use of the very therapies that saved lives the first time around.

It does seem unfair that having survived cancer once makes us likely to have it again, but that's the way it is. Cancer is currently believed to be a systemic disease, the result of a weakened immune system that permits cancers to develop. (On the other hand, the loss of immunity may be an effect rather than a cause.) The chance that you will have a recurrence or a second primary cancer is greater than the chance you had of getting the first one. The aftereffect of certain types of cancer is to become susceptible to certain other *specific* types of cancer. Breast and colon cancers, for example, develop twice as frequently in women who have had ovarian cancer as in the general population. And late-developing leukemias in longer-term survivors who have had toxic (if lifesaving) treatments with chemotherapy drugs are of increasing concern to science.

Oncology is a delicate art: Its practitioner must know how much is enough—and not too much. Most chemotherapy lowers resistance to disease because the white blood cells of the immune system are destroyed, and radiation also damages normal tissue. These effects particularly impact children in treatment. Many pediatric cancers are now considered curable, but survivors face the threat of treatment-induced secondary cancers decades ahead of them.

Finally, there is an important quality-of-life issue related to the question of five-year survival. Even within the lifetime of today's adults, cancer was a terribly wasting disease. People with cancer now are just plain healthier than they used to be. Many separate elements have contributed to a vastly improved condition:

- Effective supplemental medications that minimize treatment-induced nausea and restore vital blood and immune functions
- Better diet with more-intelligent nutritional supplementation
- Remedies for debilitating side effects like mouth sores and loss of appetite
- Effective pain control

There is nothing yet for the hair loss, which demonstrates how difficult some problems are.

People in better physical condition are better able to undergo rigorous treatment for longer periods. More people are living longer than they formerly might have, because of the development of drugs that do not kill cancer cells directly but support the health of cancer patients.

Cancer has only been considered a (somewhat) treatable disease for several decades, only a moment in the history of humanity. Its treatment has progressed remarkably, in step with impressive advances in modern medicine.

But research, based on very large population studies, is a crude system that takes little if any account of individual variation. We need treatment designed to fit our individual inner environments. Responding to the nature and degree of difference among us is the important task of science for the future. Meanwhile, it will be up to every patient (you) to ensure that the treatment you receive is the very best one you can get—for YOU.

2

CANCER TOUGH
Taking Charge

This chapter is not about specific questions of cancer treatment; it is about talking to doctors about cancer. The information they have (or have access to) about cancer can help us make treatment decisions that might affect our very lives. It becomes terribly important to ask questions effectively, in ways that will give us the most information. How should we ask those questions? And what should we ask?

"I am Oz, the Great and Terrible. Who are you, and why do you seek me?"

"I am Dorothy, the Small and Meek. I have come to you for help."
—*The Wonderful Wizard of Oz,* by L. Frank Baum

Is this any way to begin a relationship?

It's understandable, of course. Dorothy longs to return to Kansas, to the safety and comfort of home. Ordinarily a bold and spunky girl who can hold her own with witches, good or wicked, she becomes submissive and humble in the presence of Oz because she believes that only he has the power to grant her heart's desire.

Can any story be more poignantly meaningful to people with cancer? Are we not imploring the wizards of our day to use their powers to help us return "home" safely to our familiar, precancer bodies?

CANCER AS AN EMPOWERMENT ISSUE

We think of ourselves as small, frightened and made helpless by our need. We see doctors as powerful projections on a screen of our own illusions and expectations. Instead, we must learn to talk to them realistically, with the understanding that they can promise no miracles because they are (merely) people with specialized training and experience.

Since medicine became a respected profession, virtually every word on the nature of the professional relationship came from doctors who assumed it was their responsibility to make treatment decisions for you, to act as your *surrogate* in your best interest. Until our era, it was commonplace that neither patient nor family was told the true nature of a serious diagnosis. Physicians had moral authority to withhold information, especially in cancer.

MEDICAL CONSUMERISM

For anyone with the disease, there is only one priority, developing a treatment program, and only one responsibility, building a team of trusted expert advisers to help you do it. In this new era of medical consumerism, patients must become educated to the new conditions under which medical decisions are being made.

Therefore, we have to *change the way we think about ourselves* as people with cancer and to think about ourselves and our powers in a new way. Only then can we change what we expect from the health care system and change our dependency on doctors. The same tough-minded, informed decision making that we bring to buying a car or to making any other consumer purchase, we are having to apply to the purchase of medical care. We are learning to—indeed we are often *forced* to—research our own treatment options and take responsibility for the choices we make.

The symbolic change in designation from *family doctor* to the impersonal *health care provider* speaks revealingly of change in the doctor's independent role. Doctors find themselves relegated to supporting roles as our educators and advisors. As our care-driven health system becomes cost-driven, we are shifting into a more businesslike mode, even adopting the language of business: We speak of health care providers who are part of "health care delivery systems" for "medical consumers."

For the first time, we find ourselves watching television commercials for *prescription* drugs, invited by drug companies to seek our doctor's prescription for the new medication for our (self-diagnosed) condition. And medical professional organizations like the American Medical Association are lobbying patients to join them in protecting our mutual interest in health care reform because they know "you do not want patients and physicians to get lost in the system."

WHAT DO DOCTORS AND PATIENTS THINK OF EACH OTHER?

The bedrock image every patient nurtures is a doc who cares, takes care, and takes responsibility. For most of us, it's a dream. And doctors are not that sure about us either. Our attitudes toward each other have major areas of misunderstanding that lead to disappointment, ambiguous expectations, and mutual frustration.

Doctors believe that:
- We do not understand the diagnosis, and we don't hear what they are trying to tell us.
- We do not ask the right questions, which would give us the information we want.

Patients believe that:
- Wealth is an important—but concealed—priority of doctors.
- Doctors do not know how to communicate information to us.

Both patients and doctors believe that:
- The *other* person neglects the subtleties of the relationship (and both resent it).
- The *other* person acts insincerely and according to stereotyped roles.

IS COMMUNICATION REALLY A TWO-WAY STREET?

The two-way street, our long-cherished symbol of communication, has gone the way of the Model T Ford that traversed it. We're a nation of one-way streets now, which give us more efficient transportation. Perhaps we need more efficient communication, too.

The truth is, communication between patient and doctor has been more of a one-way street all along because we nonmedical types don't feel entitled to half the territory.

Doctors *expect* respect, even deference. Of course we respect their special expertise and knowledge; it's why we're there with them in the first place. And they *deserve* respect for taking on the responsibility for cutting, repairing, and healing us. Most doctors are aware of their status and depend on it to help them impress their patients. Three-fourths of the doctors surveyed by Doctor J. Alfred Jones and Gerald M. Phillips believed they were more intelligent than their patients, and nearly 100 percent of the doctors expect their patients to believe this. Sixty percent of the patients agreed.* But esteem can become reverence, and confidence can become arrogance.

We defer to doctors on a sliding scale: The more specialized and concentrated their expertise, the more likely we are to overlook what would concern us in our other relationships. We don't expect important doctors to have a bedside manner. We expect specialists to be coolly impersonal.

Yet every doctor today is a specialist. Even what were formerly GPs (general practitioners) are now FPs, specialists in family practice. For medicine in general, and cancer in particular, specialization is the nature of the practice. No doctor can possibly know everything about the details of each patient, each disease, each treatment.

Your own doctor is the one you trust enough to place at the center of a web of consultants and experts, to analyze what they have found, to convey it to you in a personal, caring manner, and to help you interpret it so that you can make informed decisions.

So much of what goes right and wrong between people has to do with the assumptions we make about the relationship when we are

---

*J. Alfred Jones and Gerald M. Phillips, *Communicating with Your Doctor* (Carbondale, IL: Southern Illinois University Press, 1988).

speaking with each other. It's helpful to become more sensitive to what's going on under the words.

THE _____ / _____
RELATIONSHIP

How would you fill in the blanks to complete _____ / _____?
Would you say "doctor/patient" or "patient/doctor"?

We customarily place the higher-status person first in conversation. Most of the time we think doctor/patient relationship, just as we think *king* and *queen*, *man* and *wife*, and, for that matter, *ham* and *eggs*. Only in power-neutral pairings, like *day* and *night* (or *night* and *day*) is no hierarchy of status suggested by the order.

When you stop to think about it, almost all conversation between people has a power relationship—or call it a *relational* relationship—underneath it. Listen to yourself, to the way *you* set up the conversation and to the assumptions *you* are making about your relationship to the other person. That listening can help you make your talk time with doctors more productive and the balance of respect between you more even. That must be your intent, or you wouldn't be reading this.

The Patient/Physician Position

Awareness of empowerment begins when we understand how we think about ourselves in relation to people, especially authorities. The real *work* of empowerment comes when we speak to them.

Dr. Eric Cassell studied doctors' responses to patients. He noticed that the first few minutes of the interaction followed the social rules we all unconsciously adhere to, the higher-status person speaking first. "The patient enters, and the doctor starts the conversation with 'Hi, how are you?' and then the patient answers. In a hospital room, however, the patient usually says the first words when the doctor comes in. This would suggest that relative social status is not the only determinant of the order of speaking. Perhaps it is a territorial matter."*

*Eric J. Cassell, *Talking with Patients* (Cambridge, MA: MIT Press, 1985), 25.

You're entitled to your own little piece of the office for the duration of the appointment. *By the action of seizing the opportunity to speak first*, even if only to introduce yourself, you announce your intention to be an activist patient. You've positioned yourself so the listener must respond to what *you* say.

Who Says What to Whom?

Now that it's established who's going to speak first, how are you going to begin? Some possibilities:

" Dr. Green, I'm Joseph Smith." *Slightly deferential, formal.*

" Dr. Green, I'm Joe Smith," or simply, "I'm Joe Smith." *More casual, friendly, but respectful.*

" Dr. Green, I'm Mr. Smith. " *Title-to-title here, clearly stating the terms.*

" Charles, I'm Joe Smith." *Don't expect groveling from me, doc!*

You get the idea. Each greeting differs in tone in small but meaningful ways because the background elements of status and social distance—all that we've learned, consciously and unconsciously, about the ways people talk to each other—affect our everyday exchanges.

Imagine how the exchange would be affected by gender, age, and racial or ethnic differences; or by wide disparities in educational or social level; or by serious physical disability. What would it mean if the patient were *Jane* Smith consulting Dr. Charles Green? Or if Jane Smith were visiting Dr. *Charlotte* Green? Or, for that matter, if *Joseph* Smith were introducing himself to Dr. Charlotte Green?

Your very first words to a doctor communicate how you see yourself in the relationship. It's your earliest opportunity to take charge. It may not come naturally at first, but it's honest and it's worth the effort.

DOING YOUR 50 PERCENT

It takes two people to make a relationship, you and your doctor. If the professional connection is important but the personal communication is not satisfactory, you can't do anything about the doctor, but *you can do something about yourself.*

The medical profession, uneasy about the unsettled nature of our relationship to each other, is devoting time to analyzing the problem in professional journals and at meetings, studying nuances of speech, nonverbal communication, and psychology—all the better to communicate with us. The least we can do is do our part to make sure the communication is effective:

Identify the problem. It's the first step in solving it.   What bothers you about what happens between you? Do you feel rushed during your appointment? You may be holding back, not getting to say what it is you really want to. If you feel there are important questions unanswered, issues undiscussed, *you* can work harder at understanding what's going on. You'll feel better and be more satisfied with the working relationship.

Feel what you're feeling.   We all bring a lot of feelings to an appointment with a doctor, from anxiety about health to irritation about waiting. Understanding what's going on can help you react appropriately so feelings don't spill over where they don't belong.

On the other hand, you may feel intimidated or inhibited from expressing what you really want to say. It's important to say what's on your mind, but a confrontation doesn't have to be confrontational. You might say something nice and disarming to pave the way, perhaps that you have complete trust in her or that you're placing yourself confidently in his hands. (Smile.) Then get to what's *really* on your mind.

Prepare for the meeting.   Go over your concerns in your mind ahead of time. Bring along your list of questions, and write down the answers, or just make notes to help you remember. Your agenda, the points you want to cover, will provide a structure for the meeting and keep both of you from straying far from the topic.

Say what you mean precisely and concisely.   The doctor is listening for specific information of a technical nature. The realities of time pressure mean that you have to speak economically. You want to use your own time efficiently also. Pare your comments to the important ones, and *don't let yourself ramble*. Ask the key questions first, then fill in with background so you don't get lost in details and storytelling.

Listen to yourself. Look at yourself. We're all so used to the sound of our own voices that we rarely stop to hear ourselves or to think about how others hear us. But other people respond to voice, tone, inflection, words.

Try to guess how you sound to the listener. It's not unusual to have a whiny, self-pitying tone if you're feeling exactly that way. But it makes it hard for doctors to sort out vague complaints from genuine symptoms because what they hear is confusing. If you sound dependent and tentative, it's difficult to be assertive. Try to stick to the hard issues: diagnosis and treatment. Don't expect a doctor to become too involved in how you feel about the disease and the problems you have because of it. There are other professionals responsible for that part of the agenda. Use them.

And the words you're using: Are they convincing, or do they convey hesitation and unsureness? You may not be sure about many things in cancer, but you should be able to be firm about your role in your own treatment. Your words reveal a lot about you and about how you see yourself in relation to the disease and to the professionals on your team. For example, did someone "send" you to see a doctor or "put" you in the hospital? Those words are better applied to a lamp than to you because they say a lot about passivity, a feeling of being an object.

Think about your body language: how you look, your posture, your expression. You've probably seen how much feeling the actors in silent films conveyed through their bodies and faces, using only minimal speech. Nonverbal communication underlines what you say in subtle and revealing ways.

Don't leave an appointment dissatisfied. If you do, it's up to you to figure out why. If you feel that the discussion has circled your real questions, try to identify what they are. Then you can say, "What I *really* want to ask is _____." Some of the longest office visits are the least productive, which means that patient and doctor both understand that something important has not been satisfied.

Don't telephone too frequently. It's perfectly natural to think of additional questions after you've left the office, and almost all doctors have telephone time set aside for that. But if you find that you telephone after your office visits *to clarify what was said* or *to add more*, you are probably not getting to what you really want to talk about during the visit.

TUNING IN

Talking to doctors is like speaking to people in a foreign country: They are likely to answer you back in their own language. So if you only know how to say what *you* want to say, you won't understand their response. And you'll miss half of what's happening between you. Conversation isn't only about talking; it's also about listening.

How to Listen

A few doctors have a wonderfully calm, attentive manner. They make you feel as if the only thing on their minds is you, and it may be, for the moment. More commonly, though, the atmosphere of activity and anxiety in a clinical setting makes things worse. Calls might interrupt your narrative, or the doctor might be paged just as you're telling where it hurts.

You can learn to develop strategies for tuning out the background noise and tuning in on what's going on between you:

Listen to the distractions. Office conditions can undermine your control and confidence. Try to identify them, then try to master them. For example, if frequent phone calls interrupt:

- Continue with the next word as if the interruption hadn't happened. That will force the doc to keep the thread of the conversation in mind (as well as you).
- Ask if calls could be held for a few minutes because this is very important to you and you'd like his or her undivided attention. Doctors are often surprised by a forthright approach from patients, but it's a businesslike thing to do and wouldn't be surprising in any other context.

Listen to body language. Be receptive to the doctor's nonverbal communication. Do you notice stolen glances at a clock? shuffling papers? fiddling with pens? Someone's trying to tell you something. Get on with your story.

On the other hand, you have a right to a respectable amount of time; so don't be intimidated. Try to find a reasonable balance.

Listen and hear.   "Listen with your fears, not your ears," says a well-known doctor. He means that we are not just a pair of ears, taking in a stream of unedited information the way a tape recorder does. Quite the opposite: Fear is a filter that keeps some information IN. We're listening *for something*, and listening very acutely.

What are we listening for (with our fears)? Bad news. When the news is good, we tend to remember it more easily. No surprise there. But anything serious that brings you to the doctor has probably put you into a state of more-or-less controlled panic. It makes it difficult to be calm. You may have to hear only one word, like *hospital* or *surgery* or *cancer*, for your mind to go blank. After that, anything of value that might be said is lost.

In an emotionally charged discussion with a doctor about your health, you may just not hear some information. Train yourself, force yourself, to listen *and* hear; or write down in your notepad the four key pieces of information you should remember. Anything else you hang onto is a bonus, and you can follow up with a call or another appointment when you have digested the initial information.

What to Listen For

All you really have to listen for is:

1. Diagnosis or hypothesis
2. Supporting evidence (reason for conclusion)
3. Suggestion of what to do next
4. Time frame

Ending Your Meeting

Don't leave the doctor's office until all loose ends are tied up.

- *Ask the doctor to confirm what was said.* When you're not *absolutely certain* you understand, "Does that mean that . . . ?" or "What does that mean?" or even "I don't understand" are perfectly reasonable responses.
- *Ask the doctor to repeat what was said* or to explain it another

way. As an experienced patient, you'll already have a notebook at hand. Make notes.

- *Make another appointment.* Ask the doctor when you should come back.
- *Review the discussion.* You may find when you are at home that you understand less than you thought at first. It takes time to get used to new ideas, especially when they are ones you and I wish we didn't have to think about.

APPOINTMENT DISAPPOINTMENT

Doctors are busy people. So are we. One of the apparently unchanging conditions of the doctor/patient relationship is that *we wait for them.* Although an appointment is an agreement that two people will meet at a certain time, who ever agreed to be the one that always waits? The unspoken message is that their time is a lot more valuable than ours because we'll wait.

Dealing with Late Appointments

The problem of waiting for doctors is one of the most vexing of the irritants that undermine our relationship—and this before we even get to see them about what's really worrying us. It's no wonder, when appointments begin in disappointment and frustration, that they frequently end up that way.

We understand that our time with them is limited and that it's not always possible to determine in advance exactly how much time each patient will require. But someone who notices that there are three names penciled into one time slot has reason to worry about how much time and attention is available. Can you do anything about it? Try these suggestions:

- *Call ahead.* Determine whether the doctor is running on schedule. If not, ask how late the schedule is running and plan your arrival accordingly.
- *Bring something to do.* Make the time you spend waiting useful.

Perhaps bring along some bills to pay, which should put you in the right frame of mind for a little discussion about appointment times.

- *Talk about the wait.* The doctor may be understanding and suggest that you schedule appointments at a certain time when the office is less busy. It may also make her or him more sensitive to the situation.
- *Consider changing doctors.* If the person can be replaced, the solution is obvious. But it might not be practical.
- *If all else fails, accept it.* Learn from the experience. It's a power struggle, and even an empowered patient can't win every time. Keep your eye on your goals.

The Ticking Clock

"My doctor just doesn't give me enough time." A common complaint. But enough time for what?

The amount of time a doctor allots to each patient must include three segments: a brief meeting (for the "What brings you here today?" question), a physical exam ("Let's have a look at you."), and an evaluation.

Too often the discussion begins at a desk, continues on the examining table, and ends up with a "by the way" question in the doorway of the office. It adds up to enough time—but doesn't feel like it.

Insist on meeting across a desk.   For both of you, it will feel more like a conference. Doctors may prefer to talk in scattered sound bites because it's more economical use of their time, but you have every right to say that you will feel more comfortable working this way. Mention that a structured discussion is more efficient because you will not have to call with questions. (Then don't.)

Pin down loose ends.   Ask what day to telephone for test results. Ask when to make the next appointment for treatment. It's in your interest to ask specific questions when the doctor is most focused on you and your case, not when another patient is the priority or when yours is just one telephone call in a busy day.

HOW INVOLVED DO YOU
WANT TO BE?

More critical than any question you might ask is letting your doctor know *to what degree you want to participate* in your own medical decision making. There are two concerns:

Responsibility

How much responsibility do you want? The doctor should be receptive to clues from you about *your* expectations. How much do you want to participate in the decision-making process? in discussing the options? in researching new treatment possibilities? You can shape the relationship by the questions you ask, indicating your interest in expanding your own knowledge and involvement.

Technical Data

How much technical data can you comfortably handle? Some diagnostic tests have advanced to a point where they can identify prognostic (predictive) factors relatively accurately—without being able to do anything about them. Not everyone will be comfortable with *that* information—if a patient thinks he or she stands less chance of winning, it could undermine the will to fight.

Can the degree of technical analysis available undermine *your doctor's* determination or ability to do everything possible for you? Be alert to the possibility. Managed-care plans and health insurers may *require* your oncologist to limit treatment if they believe from the indicators that your chances of beating the disease are diminished. If you sense hesitation or think you are being denied treatment, you have both practical and legal recourse. (See Chapter 7.)

Fear of Feeling

We're at a disadvantage when discussing our health with physicians because they are trained to be unemotional and unreactive, and we are not. (And it *is* our health at risk!)

Physicians use scientific, technical, and anatomical terms because:

• They are trained to do so.
• The terms are neutral and impersonal.
• The terms are precise, exactly describing specific medical conditions.

Physicians' detachment from your emotional state allows them to evaluate appropriate treatment recommendations without the bias of emotional involvement. It also helps them keep their own pity and fear at a distance. When doctors talk about your illness, their use of language reinforces that detachment, as if saying, "We're talking about a diseased organ system here, not a person." But it can be *felt* as isolating to the patient, who is powerfully aware of one thing: "It's *me* we're talking about!"

Doctors fear that their patients will become emotional. They avoid having to deal with emotion by creating an environment that's unreceptive to its expression. Withdrawing from the feeling level of communication into a professional response, they react impersonally. When patients weep or become teary—which happens—it sets up a conventional scenario that may lead both patient and doctor into misleading, patterned responses. And because everyone feels awkward when other adults cry, it may evoke the kind of paternalistic response that is disempowering, just what you don't want. Louise, a determined young Californian undergoing treatment for a gynecological cancer, shared her experience: "I'm a crier. When I start to cry, I say to my doctor, 'Don't think that just because I'm crying, anything is different. I can't help the tears—it's an emotional reaction. But I'm just as tough crying as not crying!' And I go on talking right through the tears."

Reacting emotionally to the important things you're discussing is not in itself a problem. *How you act on it, though, is your choice.* Most men don't cry because they feel it is not manly, whereas the range of acceptable behavior open to women has more latitude. The act of expressing emotion itself need not stop the progress of treatment or the acquisition of knowledge. The message you want to give is, "I'm *feeling* this way about a problem, so let's discuss what we're going to *do* about it."

THE THREE MOST FREQUENTLY ASKED QUESTIONS NOT TO ASK

There are no satisfactory answers to the three most common questions patients ask of doctors. Asking them places you both in an awkward position, because the questions may disguise underlying emotional concerns.

1. *"If I were a member of your family, what treatment would you recommend?"*

When treatment decisions must be made in what is usually an emotionally stressful situation, some people, particularly women, are likely to ask this question. But it's not a good question to ask because:

- Most doctors, appropriately, will not respond directly to what really is an indirect appeal to their emotions. You're *not* a member of the family. The question suggests that they would withhold the best treatment information from their patients, yet physicians as a group have serious professional pride that suggests the opposite is true.
- It's a no-win question. One hematologist answers his most-asked question by saying that he treats *every* patient like a member of his family. It's a thoughtful response, but not what you want to hear. To you it could feel like an evasion.
- It might not be in your best interests. Emotional bias can affect treatment decisions *adversely*, although the question assumes the opposite is true.
- No doctor *can* answer it objectively. The best treatment for someone else may not be the best treatment for *you* because of the nature of the illness or the personality of the patient. Someone else may have different values or perhaps be more (or less) inclined to accept medical authority without question or to accept more (or less) aggressive treatment.

It's a question that begs to be patronized, can never have a satisfactory answer, and can only leave you feeling disempowered. But a related question to ask, one that is ever more pressing, is, "If *insurance coverage* weren't the issue, what would you recommend?"

2. *"What are my chances, Doc?"*

One of the conversational dead ends with which you *don't* want to start a discussion is the one that most people will use to do just that. It appears to be a simple request for specific information; but it doesn't come right out and directly ask, "What will happen to me?"

If you ask your doctor what your chances of surviving cancer are, you'll probably get an answer to the *explicit* question, a statistical answer like "one in three" or "sixty percent." But is that what you want to know? Any answer that falls short of "One hundred percent long-term survival, guaranteed!" is going to sound less than encouraging—at that moment, anyway.

"Chances" are statistics. There are two facts you have to know about statistics:

- *They can only suggest what the experience of any individual patient might be.* Data is numerical information based on the experience of large numbers of people and is *only* applicable to groups. You usually cannot tell where you will fall in the statistics.
- *They are based on data collected some time ago from studies that were done some time before that.* No matter how current and meaningful statistics try to be, they are always somewhat out of date. *Your* treatment profile and survival are going to provide data for newer statistics, which is being gathered right now. *You* are data.

Statistics are a *guide* to evaluating treatment plans. Your treatment choices may be different from what was available to people whose treatment outcomes provided the data. Given progress in research and the number and variety of clinical trials for cancer, you may have the opportunity to be treated with newer drugs or technology *for which incomplete or no comparable statistics exist.* An experienced professional could be asked for an evaluation of *possibilities.* If certain treatment regimens are known or even thought to be more effective in prolonging survival or offering the possibility of cure, it is surely something you want to know.

3. *"How long do you give me?"*

The crystal-ball questions—"How long do you give me" or, its variant, "How long do I have?"—are about time. Or are they?

On the surface, they request a simple answer from a professional, familiar with the expected course of the disease. But these questions are not about time any more than the previous one was a question about numbers. They're about what will happen.

For most of us, our own diagnosis is our first encounter with the disease. We are inexperienced, naive in its ways. We depend upon the experts' knowledge of the disease and its treatment, asking for a prediction based on that expertise. But it takes experience to learn that nothing about cancer is predictable. During the time Louise was in chemotherapy, her oncologist's father died of cancer. Louise observed, "He couldn't do a thing for him. It showed me a lot about the limitations on a doctor's powers."

Nevertheless, an experienced professional should be asked for an evaluation of *possibilities*. If certain treatment regimens are known to be or are even thought to be more effective in prolonging survival or offering the possibility of cure, it is surely something you want to know.

Clinical evaluations of new medications involve the largest possible number of patients in order to observe whether therapies are beneficial. *Individual variations in response are lost in the process.* So physicians cannot simply tell you how much time *you* have. And they cannot foresee the future.

On the other hand, should you ask about time, get an answer, and then outlive the prediction, you'll feel as if you've really beaten the odds (or evaded the baleful eye of Fate). When Fred Lebow, president of the New York Road Runners Club, died in late 1994, radio announcers reported, "When he was diagnosed with brain cancer in 1992, his doctors gave him six months to live."

Living with Uncertainty

Aren't questions about time and statistics asking a great-and-powerful someone for something that no one can grant? It's not a crystal-ball vision that's being asked for, not a prediction of the future, and certainly not just time. It's a moving request for life. And no one, unfortunately, has that much power.

What you can do: *Learn to live with uncertainty.* There are few certainties in this complex illness. Cancer treatment is a long-term process; and, at the end of it, there's still no absolute resolution, just because it's cancer.

Value today. No one knows what will happen tomorrow. And we can't change either day very much, anyway.

MONEY: THE BOTTOM LINE

In these days of let-it-all-hang-out openness, the only taboo left may be talking about money. And if fee-for-service medical care goes the way of modesty, it won't be a problem much longer.

But until then, it could happen that, while your doctor is talking to you about your condition, you're thinking about what this visit (consultation, tests, follow-up, and maybe more) is costing you. You are probably reluctant to bring it up, even though you're uneasy or distressed by financial concerns.

Money is an obstacle in the medical relationship. Patients generally believe that doctors' fees are too high, and they resent contributing to a lifestyle in a socioeconomic bracket higher than their own. As a result, patients as a group are unsympathetic to the economic pressures on the medical profession.

As the pressure for change intensifies, patients who are urged to become skilled participants in medical decision making are finding that doctors are spending *less* time with them and giving less care. So what can you do if you have a billing problem?

Don't be embarrassed. Talk about it. Most doctors today have a staff that handles billing and accounting. If there are fee problems, start there. But don't hesitate to talk to your doctor very frankly about your concerns because it's unlikely that the office staff has set the billing policies.

Find out who is responsible for a problem. Identify where the problem originates, which may be the managed-care plan, insurer, or other provider. If so, you can shift your attention to them.

Be a consumer. Keep costs down. Ask about generic drugs, which are *often* (not always) less expensive and equally effective substitutes for more expensive ones still under patent and protected from competitive market forces on price. Or suggest that it might be sufficient to start with one diagnostic test, instead of a complete series, because it can be followed stepwise if necessary. Although constraints on physicians have contributed to slowing the rise in health care costs, it's part of *your* empowerment to communicate that you know that some economies are in your interest, also.

Talk to your insurer about ways to maximize the extent of your coverage. Your direct involvement may be persuasive. All organizations have patient representatives. Explain that you are trying to be a responsible medical consumer and that your goals are the same as theirs, economical use of the system.

Work to ensure quality care. Patients need protection from those who would abuse the system. We hear of insurers that process paper without ever looking at what's written on it and of medical providers who overprescribe tests when they own the diagnostic hardware. Nevertheless, many people have been frustrated when they've sought responsible correction of the system. Congress has evaded its responsibility so far. Quality-of-care issues are bound to become more prominent as managed care becomes more prevalent.

In many individual states, associations of voluntary health organizations have formed ad hoc committees to ensure that the quality of health care services will not be compromised. More people need to be involved. If you are thinking, "I'm just one person—what can *I* do?" such a committee may be where you can contribute to making things better for yourself and others. (See Chapter 9.)

RECOGNIZING THE VOCABULARY OF VICTIMIZATION—AND WHAT TO DO ABOUT IT

Empowerment is a *process of increasing awareness that leads to a sense of one's own possibilities.* Recognizing the meaning and message in words gives you control over how you use them and how you permit others to use them around you. And the language of cancer could certainly use some empowerment. Consider the following:

Sticks and Stones

When we hear about *suffering* cancer patients or *victims* of cancer, we should recognize that those words *weaken and undermine the patients and their empowerment.* Victims are people who are badly treated, who suffer or are oppressed by their passivity or through no fault of their own. Society pities victims and patronizes them.

This attitude was displayed by the producer of a daytime TV show: "I'm looking for cancer victims to be in the audience for _____'s show next Tuesday. Can your group send some people?" When asked if she was looking for "patients," the producer replied "Well, I've always thought of people with cancer as victims. There are some cancer victims in my own family, and *they* don't seem to mind."

Allowing others to define us to ourselves is the ultimate *dis*empowerment. When everyone thinks of people with cancer as victims, can we help thinking about ourselves that way? The word *victim* implies a permanent condition, unless you've ever heard of a "temporary victim." It's time to get rid of the persistent association with weakness and suffering.

Cancer as Metaphor

Cancer is the biggest linguistic bomb we can drop.

John Dean, counsel to President Nixon, hinting at the nature of the events of the Watergate break-in, warned "There is a cancer on the presidency. . . ."

Cancer as a metaphor, representing utter disaster, contaminates our speech and taints our thoughts. We all get the message, and frankly, it's cancer as worst-case scenario. *Malignant, metastatic, spreading like cancer*—all these terms convey images of relentless, insidious evil when they're used in nonmedical contexts.

It's a cheap shot. Do you think of yourself as the personification of the most awful thing that can happen? Probably not! Yet that's the image in people's minds when they think about *you* having cancer. It's our national cancer-image problem. We internalize images of negativity, and they're hard to get rid of.

What can you do about it? Plenty! Whenever you see or hear *cancer* used to describe something terrible, speak up! Write to a newspaper or magazine, or contact the source of the remark and, politely but firmly explain that it is offensive, that they should be aware of why it is, and that they should please stop! It's an empowering step for you and (maybe) an empowering *stop* for them.

The Long-, Long-suffering Patient

"So-and-so suffered from cancer for six years." How often have you read this uncomfortable turn of phrase? Probably so frequently that you don't even notice anything wrong with it—it seems normal.

Of course, people *do* suffer from cancer in many ways. But they also suffer greatly from other things, like bursitis, a notoriously painful inflammation of shoulder or knee joints. Yet if you were to read, "So-and-so suffered from housemaid's knee for six years," you'd automatically recognize that *suffered* in that context is being used in the figurative sense—it means "*had* housemaid's knee." ("Housemaid's knee" is an old name for bursitis.)

Saying "so-and-so suffered" taps into everyone's fear that the word is being used literally. *Cancer* and *suffering* are an insufferable combination, speechwise.

In Rem

Have you ever heard people, speaking of their own cancer treatment, say that they are "in remission"? If so, did they sound euphoric, thrilled, or even very, very happy? Or did you catch an edge of anxiety in the words?

If ever a word had a grey cloud hanging above it, *remission* is it. Remission is a *lessening in the severity* of symptoms or the *temporary disappearance* of symptoms during the course of an illness. Note the hedge words, *lessening* and *temporary*. We're not talking cure here; we're not even talking hope.

Remission is a convenient term used by physicians to denote the period between one time when a cancer is active and the next time, when it returns or progresses—a doomsday scenario that I, for one, don't buy into. Speaking of cure may be unrealistic, given the uncertainty of cancer treatment; but if the cancer is in remission, at least you can hope it's not absolutely, positively coming back.

You have the power to choose how you speak about yourself. There are no other words available to describe that period when your treatment is finished, no synonyms for *remission* to offer more hope or to admit of other possible outcomes. You have your entire future ahead of you; and there you are under a little cloud of "remission," when your goal is to be free of cancer.

Nevertheless, it's useful or necessary sometimes to describe just where you are in the ongoing process of cancer. What can you say instead?

1. "*I'm* fine. And the cancer's in remission."
2. "I'm out of treatment for X years (or months.)" *Out of treatment* is a way of stating exactly where you are, without getting into predicting the future and without inferring that you're scanning the landscape for the recurrence that could come along any day now.
3. "I'm finished with treatment." Even if it's only for now, it's a simple statement of fact.

A Bout with Cancer

You might get the idea that fighting cancer is sport if you read about people who went down for the count:

> Benner passed away in June 1990 at age 44, after *a long bout* with malignant melanoma, but the program he launched continues . . .*
> John B_____ died on July 15, 1990, after *a bout* with cancer.†

Why do we have such a hard time talking about cancer? The boxing metaphor at least is suitable: There are several rounds to go before the fight is won or lost. It hurts. And, most important, boxers are fighters. But cancer doesn't fight fairly or play by rules. Talking about *having* cancer is reality; talking about a bout with cancer trivializes it, makes it a bit of a game.

---

*Charles Bowen and David Peyton, *How to Get the Most Out of CompuServe*, 5th ed. (New York: Random House, 1993).

†Obituary, *New York Times*, 20 October 1994.

Fighting cancer is both physical and emotional, but the fight for empowerment is a bout with ideas that confine and constrain us. Facing the disease directly enables us to deal with reality directly. It's one thing to deliberately challenge its power by saying mockingly, "I had a bout with cancer." It's quite another for an obituary to employ that image.

Alias Cancer

Cancer has been called a lot of things over the centuries, including "buboes," possibly the untamed ancestor of our own childish "boo-boos."

But even today, not everyone calls cancer by its name. People who speak of another's disease frequently refer to it as C-A, their voices dropping to a whisper, perhaps in fear of attracting the disease to themselves. *And so do doctors*.

Medical charts, notorious for bearing an alphabet soup of abbreviations, commonly show the notation "C-A." Who has not heard cancer called The Big C or The Big One, as if mocking the magnitude of the disease diminishes the power it has over us? Using aliases disguises the real nature of the disease and pushes away the fear felt by patients and physicians alike.

Professionals should not communicate their own fear to us because we are looking for (unconscious) reassurance that they are more powerful than the cancer. When doctors use euphemisms, they show that they too are afraid of the real words and real concepts, like *disease* and *death*.

Fighting for your life is a real-world event. *If you have cancer, don't be afraid to say so.* Calling any disease by its name implies that there is knowledge about it and that there is something to do about it. It's demystified. It's just another disease.

3

GETTING INFORMATION ON TREATMENT OPTIONS AND CHOICES

S tartling changes in the ways we think of ourselves in relationship to health care professionals are at hand, and treatment options may never be the same. It was electronic communication that brought ALS (the debilitating neuromuscular disease known as Lou Gehrig's disease) patients and advocates together over an urgent issue not unlike the one that often confronts the cancer community: the need for faster response from health and regulatory authorities. Substantial anecdotal evidence suggested that a drug approved for use for a different condition could also be effective for treating some people with ALS. Because the number of people with ALS is small, realistically, there is little incentive for the drug's manufacturer to do the research necessary to secure FDA approval. The widely scattered (but highly motivated) ALS on-line group raised funds to sponsor research that is expected to demonstrate the drug's therapeutic effect. If that happens, you can be sure that patients will drive the drug toward FDA approval so that it will be covered by health insurers. Think about the possibilities of patients sponsoring targeted research! When knowledgeable, committed people are able to break through business-as-usual mental barriers, almost anything can happen.

Only a few years ago, we weren't even in the ballpark when it came to researching treatments for our own diseases. By making access to medical libraries difficult for nonprofessionals, the medical establishment effectively barred us from the literature or original sources of information. Patients were expected to be passive recipients of medical services.

Now there's a whole new picture—and it's appearing on our computer screens. With no intention of providing unlimited information *directly* to the public, the National Cancer Institute (NCI) has done exactly that in the process of servicing medical and commercial users. The Cancer Information Service (CIS) was established to be the conduit for transmitting selected information from the Physician's Data Query (PDQ) by telephone and mail to patients. But the information superhighway has turned out to have far more exit ramps than NCI imagined, many of them leading directly to our own front doors. And advocates, consumer groups, and commercial interests have stepped right through in order to reach us directly.

As we realize how much information is available to us and learn how to get it and use it (and as it gets easier to use), we are putting pressure on the health care system to "include us in." We have been marginalized, kept out of policy loops in issues of importance to us. But it won't be easy to shut out a generation of informed medical consumers. The FDA cannot long deny access to useful new therapies when large numbers of people know about them, know how to get them, and consider it their *right* to have them.

The amount of information you collect can quickly become overwhelming. It should be organized as it accumulates. A loose-leaf notebook is a sensible place to keep the material. Divide it into sections so you can efficiently find and refer to what you need. You'll need sections for your medical history (make chronological entries of your tests, treatments, and consultations), information you collect, for organization newsletters, and for names of contacts. Keep sheets of blank paper in each section for your own notes. Highlight key words in your collected literature in brightly colored marker (the neon colors are great) so you can quickly spot what the paper is about.

MEDICALINGO

Medicalingo, the vocabulary and usage of health care professionals, is a Rosetta stone, the key to understanding and participating in medical communication and decision making. You may feel uncomfortable with medicalingo at first; but you don't need to go to medical school in order to understand it and to use it with confidence. Can you learn that *renal* translates as kidney and *hepatic* as liver? Trust me: You can.

Why Medical Terms?

When you talk to members of the medical profession, it makes sense to know and use medical terms because

- Medical terms are very precise. When you speak about a diagnosis, a part of your body, or a treatment effect, you and the doctor both know *exactly* what you're talking about.
- Medical terms give you emotional distance. After all, it's *your* body you're talking about. Doctors are professionally detached from your feelings about your condition, and it's useful to adopt a little of that for yourself so you can discuss your health unemotionally.
- Medical terms give you credibility with your physicians. Professionals will take you more seriously when they respect you and the effort you've demonstrably made to meet them halfway.

How to Learn Medicalingo

Build your own medical library.   A medical dictionary and a reference book of medical terminology will be great assets to you. Look up new words, terms, and descriptions as you read them in order to deepen your knowledge. Having references at hand helps.

Write down the meanings of new terms.   Most people remember things better when they are written down. While you do it, you'll be developing a very selective and personal glossary of terms from the medical literature. Get to recognize prefixes, such as *exo-* (outside of) and *endo-* (within), and suffixes such as *-tomy* (a surgical incision, as in *gastrectomy*) and *-scopy* (examining or observing through an instrument, as in *gastroscopy*).

Make sure you know the names of drugs of interest to you.   Each of them has a scientific name and a trade name (e.g., paclitaxel—

Taxol; docetaxel—Taxotere; cyclophosphamide—Cytoxan). In reports about treatment regimens, drug combinations are often referred to by their initials or acronyms; for example, CAF (used for breast cancer) involves use of Cytoxan, Adriamycin, and 5-FU.

You also have to become familiar with the combinations you are following, because they can be confusing: A, for example, can stand for both doxorubicin (Adriamycin) *and* dactinomycin (Actinomycin D). Both C and CTX can refer to Cytoxan. And in the CHOP regimen for non-Hodgkin's lymphoma, it's the H that stands for doxorubicin.

If there are multiple protocols for the type of disease you are researching, make a good clear reference list of the drugs on each regimen and what their initials stand for so you get to know them.

Collect popular articles. Every public library has the *Readers' Guide to Periodical Literature*, an index to articles appearing in consumer magazines and nontechnical journals, and most also have electronic retrieval systems. When topics like breast cancer or prostate cancer or insurance problems receive a lot of coverage in the press, skilled journalists may produce a rich variety of articles that will give you a thorough introduction to and some background on those topics. Look up and make copies of articles that you find helpful.

YOUR FIRST AND FASTEST RESOURCE: CANCERFAX

Almost everyone's first impulse when diagnosed with cancer is to telephone *someone* for help. It's the right idea, but there's a brand new wrinkle: Make the call from a fax/phone. The NCI service called CancerFax can give you easy, immediate access to a huge amount of information in its PDQ (Physician's Data Query) database. PDQ is a national central repository of electronic information about cancer. The database contains (1) all the medical information about your disease that you can use; (2) clinical trials in which NCI participates; (3) news and reports on cancer diagnosis, treatment, and prevention; and (4) CANCERLIT citations and abstracts, which summarize the newest research published in the past six months for about eighty types of cancer. When you speak with specialists at the CIS, they are themselves searching PDQ for information to give you. CancerFax makes it available to you directly, twenty-four hours a day, seven days a week.

How to Use CancerFax

1. *From the fax/phone*, dial 1-301-402-5874. This will connect you to the CancerFax computer in Bethesda, Maryland.
2. You will be asked to choose between English and Spanish. Enter the number (1 for English, 2 for Spanish). Then you are voice-welcomed to the CancerFax system and offered instructions for proceeding and a menu of choices. If you are a first-time user, select the complete fifteen-page CancerFax Contents, which includes the list of six-digit code numbers that you will need to identify the type of cancer and the reports you're interested in having. *You need the entire list.* There's a wealth of information available, but you must know the codes. (If you already have the list, skip to 4, below.) Should you make a mistake, press the 0 (zero) key to start over.
3. When you have the Contents, make a second call to request the PDQ Patient Statement for the type of cancer in which you are interested. (Each request requires a separate call; you cannot get back into the system afterward.) Every PDQ Statement for a type of cancer has two six-digit code numbers: one beginning with 200- for patients and a *separate* one starting with 100- for medical professionals. You may request either statement, depending on your knowledge and the level of technical information you want. The patient information is thorough but basic, written so it can be understood by people who may have a wide variation in educational background. It's an excellent place to start. Note that only the PDQ Statements have separate tracks; everything else has only one code number.
4. A voice will confirm the information you've selected and tell you how many pages will be transmitted. Press the 1 key to confirm or the 0 (zero) key to cancel if there is any error.
5. You will be prompted to press START/COPY or RECEIVE on your fax machine and then to hang up the phone. The transmission will begin.

What You Can Get from CancerFax

The complete printout begins with clear instructions for accessing the service, followed by a Contents list with all the six-digit reference numbers. There are four types of information available:

PDQ Statements   Information about the selected cancer, written either for patients or for health care professionals. Patients receive a description, diagnostic indications, staging information, and updated treatment options, and are offered some related NCI publications and a referral to the 800-4-CANCER telephone number to speak with an information specialist. Physicians get a highly detailed analysis of the disease and its standard treatment, as well as an indication of treatments under clinical evaluation, with references to the medical literature.

Supportive-care information is included (300- code numbers), which covers health problems caused by the disease and its treatment that patients commonly experience, such as fatigue, mouthsores, and sleep disorders. Information on other topics can be accessed with separate code numbers—topics like screening and prevention (300- code numbers), clinical trials (400- code numbers), and news of especially noteworthy investigational or newly approved drugs (800- code numbers).

CancerFax News   Information about what is available on the PDQ database and how to connect directly to it. Many large medical centers and some university and public libraries have access to PDQ, and NCI licenses several companies to distribute the information commercially. Between what's available through CancerFax and the CIS, you may not need to access PDQ yourself; but if you want to, NCI tells you how. The 400- code numbers provide information about NCI resources, programs, and publications. There are also instructions for reaching PDQ via the Internet (CancerNet).

CancerFax has a Bulletin section that reproduces important current studies, papers, or articles. There is no charge for use of those services that do not involve a commercial distributor (although some do). Note that the code numbers change frequently, so you must use a current Contents to obtain the report(s) you want. Instead of printing out fifteen pages again, however, you can update a fairly current CancerFax by requesting document number 405001, which details changes made to PDQ summaries since the last update, or document 400000, which will give information on changes in Fact Sheets.

NCI Fact Sheets   Publications from the Office of Cancer Communication at NCI, the public relations arm of NCI, about clinical and public policy issues of cancer (600- code numbers). These papers must be read (in the author's opinion) with a great deal of skepticism. In such diverse reports as "Artificial Sweeteners," "In Answer to Your Questions about Agent Orange," and "Personal Use of Hair Coloring Products and Risk of Cancer," the NCI generally communicates information from a very safe—and very uninformative—position, as if its role were that of quieting public concerns about cancer. Consider the following passage:

> Industrial and environmental carcinogens often act with other agents or with certain factors in an individual to cause cancer. In addition, a large proportion of all cancers are related to the use of tobacco and to things we eat and drink.*

Except for smoking, the NCI virtually never suggests that anything specific can cause cancer, even though a not-insignificant portion of the NCI budget is dedicated to research into the cause and prevention of cancer. Can the information from Fact Sheet 600032 help you avoid carcinogenic substances? Obviously it cannot, even though there are hundreds of known carcinogens besides tobacco, carcinogens that get into our bodies and can start the process of cancer.

Understand what kind of problem would be created for health authorities if some common, everyday substances or environmental conditions were proven to cause cancer. Subtle pressure exists to minimize those eventualities. It's the same problem as the use of mass screening to detect various cancers: NCI rejects it as not "cost-effective" because relatively few cases would be found *in the general population*, even though you or I might benefit from having a cancer

---

*National Cancer Institute, "Tests for Carcinogenicity," NCI Fact Sheet 600032.

detected early. NCI takes too lofty and detached a position on many issues when it should be our advocate, advancing our interests in prevention and control of cancer.

CANCERLIT   A cancer-specific database, arranged by topic, of the contents of approximately 4,000 medical journals worldwide, reports of meetings and symposia, and selected monographs (in-depth reports on a single subject). The information, dating back to 1978, consists of citations (which refer you to the original publication for the entire article) and abstracts (brief summaries of the purpose, experimental method, and conclusions of the study). Although foreign publications are not generally available in English, the abstracts are usually translated, so the information is accessible. Codes and instructions are provided in the CancerFax transmission.

What to Do Next

After you have studied the fifteen-page CancerFax Contents, decide which reports you will request. Redial the CancerFax number, then (at the voice prompt) enter the six-digit code number for the PDQ Statement you want.

Having studied the Statement printout about your disease and any other material of interest to you, you may be curious about or ready for the more difficult material of the health care professionals' Statements. These also contain a bibliography, so you can look up an original article in its entirety.

When you have read the information from PDQ, whether patient, professional, or both, you should have a good, clear, better-than-basic understanding of your disease and of both standard treatment and promising new treatments.

It's useful to follow that reading with a selective reading of the CANCERLIT abstracts. You will become familiar with standard and new drugs in various experimental combinations and with the results. You'll notice that often the literature contains reports that *no* effectiveness has been found with certain drugs—useful information to have.

When you have absorbed all the information you've requested and understand the nature of and questions about your type of cancer, you're ready for the next step.

YOUR NEXT RESOURCE: 1-800-4-CANCER

The Cancer Information Service provides much helpful information, but you can use it most productively when you know what to ask for. To speak with an information specialist at CIS, call 1-800-4-CAN-CER.

The CIS has nineteen regional offices nationwide to serve the public, including medical professionals, which are open Monday through Friday, 9 A.M. to 7 P.M., except for federal holidays. (Try calling either early or late to avoid the usually busy times.) Specialists proficient in languages other than English may be available, depending on the need in different regions.

The CIS can answer questions about diagnosis and treatment, smoking-cessation programs, and clinical trials. They have directories of medical specialists, institutions, and organizations involved in care, treatment, and support. The person with whom you speak will ask you specifics about your case and treatment to match your needs to the options available. Have your notes with you, and list your questions in advance so you are sure of getting them all answered.

ON-LINE: THE INFORMATION REVOLUTION IN CANCER

If you are computer knowledgeable and have the time, the modem, and the money, you can access a great deal of information.

Using Software

Computer software offers the simplest packages of electronic health information you can find. Useful, well-known medical reference books, like *The Mayo Clinic Family Health Book*, are available, often in interactive (CD-ROM) versions. Many others are in preparation, books such as medical dictionaries and guides to symptoms, surgery, treatment (the Merck Manual), and prescription and nonprescription drugs (a consumer software version of the *Physician's Desk Refer-*

ence, the famed PDR). A CD for Windows called *Family Health Tracker* (published by Great Bear/HealthSoft) provides a practical electronic notebook in which to keep track of your medical history, including drugs and doses. You must be methodical about using it, though; it cannot automatically enter each treatment for you—yet.

MEDLARS

The National Library of Medicine (NLM) in Maryland maintains several on-line databases known collectively as MEDLARS, some parts of which are confusing because of their similar names and content (MEDLARS, MEDLINE, GRATEFUL MED). It includes some material available in the same form through other media and also some unique information:

• MEDLINE, a computer compilation of several authoritative indexes formerly available primarily in medical libraries, gives you access to more than 7 million citations and abstracts drawn from 4,000 American and foreign publications, both well-known and obscure, concerned with medicine, surgery, dentistry, nursing, and health care management.
• CANCERLIT (See p. 64.)
• PDQ, a database of many parts has, besides the detailed PDQ Statements (see p. 62), reports on NCI clinical trials; detection, screening, and prevention information; and directories of institutions and physicians specializing in cancer treatment.
• TOXLINE and TOXLIT consist of 2 million reference databases of toxicology citations about the effects of drugs and other chemicals. This information is of special interest because it does not seem to be available anywhere else.
• RTECS, the computerized Registry of Toxic Effects of Chemical Substances, has information about more than 117,000 potentially toxic substances.
• HEALTH is a database of more than a half million citations to literature on health care planning and delivery, insurance, financial management, and related topics.
• CHID, the Combined Health Information Database, was developed by agencies of the U.S. Public Health Service. It contains citations and references to a wide range of health material intended

for use by the public as well as professionals and educators. You can access CHID through BRS Online, an authorized vendor; call CHID's customer service at 1-800-289-4BRS for information and costs, or find it at many medical, university, or public libraries.

• GRATEFUL MED is software from the National Library of Medicine (NLM) that will give you access to NLM databases, including the important PDQ clinical trial protocols (the same database from which the CIS selects trials when you call them) and CANCERLIT (the database of current medical abstracts).

Although you can purchase GRATEFUL MED from the NLM, CancerNet and on-line computer services have outpaced the need for it. Some medical libraries have the software program, which may be available for your use.

The NLM staff can help individuals search any of the MEDLARS databases. For information about NLM programs and services, call the Office of Public Information, Monday through Friday, 8:30 A.M. to 5 P.M. (Eastern time) at 1-800-272-4787 or 301-496-6308. Or call the MEDLARS Management Desk at 1-800-638-8480 to arrange to have a search done.

Commercial On-line Services

You can reach other people to exchange information and cancer experience by using commercial on-line services. Depending on your time and involvement, you can choose just to get your toes wet (receive e-mail about a special interest) or to plunge right into the cyberwave by joining a newsgroup or by participating in direct, real-time electronic interaction with others.

The services have a wealth of general medical forums: There are "wellness" forums, medical references, and health hotlines of many kinds. Note that there are surcharges above basic service costs for some of the forums, particularly those that get you into specialized databases. Using message centers (in which you post queries and collect answers at your own convenience) puts you in touch with (literally) countless other people who have had a variety of medical experiences. The level of give-and-take in the discussions can be high, depending on the participants and the systems operator who mediates the interaction. It's not uncommon for doctors to join in, and people on-line tend to be very supportive. Not only is it possible that someone will be able to help you, but you may find that your own experiences can help others. Do exercise some caution, though: *You do not know the background, credentials, or biases of the people whose opinions are offered.*

What You Can Find On-line

CompuServe has a rich offering of services related to cancer. They have HealthNet, a general medical reference with introductory-level information about cancer (and other diseases); Cancer Forum, in which you can exchange information and support; and Comprehensive Core Medical Library (CCM), a search service of the Massachusetts Medical Society. For an additional charge, you can look up original journal articles that you might have come across as references in your other readings. (GO PDQ) will get you into NCI's PDQ database, which gives you via computer much of the information available through CancerFax and more, including a 12,000-name list of cancer specialists. PaperChase (GO PAPERCHASE) gives you access to MEDLINE and other informative databases. Call CompuServe at 1-800-848-8990.

America Online (AOL) provides many similar services and also offers the American Cancer Society Forum, which contains software libraries of its own publications that you can download immediately. All the services offer Internet access, but at present their capabilities vary, a situation sure to even out within a short period of time. With the Net you can easily reach such exotic repositories of cutting-edge scientific information as the National Cancer Center in Japan. Call America Online at 1-800-827-6364.

Prodigy has a medical-support bulletin board for many different diseases, among which is cancer (jump: HEALTH BB). Members often set up their own "chat room" for continuing discussions, and doctors are available to answer on-line queries. Although this service does not presently offer access to medical libraries, Prodigy has a "Homework Helper," which locates articles in the popular press based on key words you choose. Call Prodigy at 1-800-776-3449.

Because the growth of on-line services and bulletin boards has been tumultuous, it has also been haphazard. There is no central directory or means of locating the diverse bulletin boards and no way of knowing what one service offers compared with another. You can and should take a trial (often free) membership in a commercial service to see what it offers before you become a permanent subscriber. Some diligent clicking will give you a sense of what value a service has for you.

Sponsored and Special-Interest Bulletin Boards

Many health organizations, hospitals, and institutions maintain their own bulletin board systems (BBSs) for posting information or receiving and responding to queries from consumers via modem. The National Kidney Cancer Association BBS, for instance, makes 700 files of information, including the latest kidney cancer clinical trials, available 24 hours a day, toll-free, seven days a week. Call 1-800-280-2032 for instructions.

The American Cancer Society has a BBS at 219-864-2502. Black Bag, a general medical BBS, also has extensive cancer information. Call 610-454-7396 to sign on.

The difficulty lies in finding what's out there. A BBS can be on the Internet or in any of the commercial on-line services, or it can be freestanding (dialed directly). If you think an organization has a BBS, call the organization to learn how the BBS can be accessed.

The Internet

The Internet, the global computer network, may become the means of finally knitting the fragmented cancer-patient base into a "virtual community." Right now, we are a two-layered society—one layer, the people who know how to navigate the still-shapeless Internet; and the other layer, all the rest of us. It's safe to predict that we'll be in touch with each other in entirely new ways in the future.

Patients already consulting with each other share knowledge of their experiences. Now with images of your own or reference cancers easily transmissible, long-distance consultations will likely become commonplace. Much more data will be accessible to deepen the level of knowledge. You'll be able to compare doctors' expertise and training, as well as their track records with specific types of cancer. The same correlations can be made for hospitals, so you'll be sure you're going to the most experienced people or facilities, which could be critically important if you are having a relatively new procedure or therapy. Many important cancer centers are already developing "Home Pages" that offer to Internet users extensive information, case histories, and references.

As the Internet inevitably becomes more systematized, it will be easier to find information, services, and each other. And as it inevitably becomes commercialized, we, too, will be easier to find. Pharmaceutical manufacturers will be able to reach their end-market (you, the consumer) by establishing World Wide Web sites containing information that you want to know but presently find difficult to get. One example is the "indigent drug programs," through which manufacturers provide treatment drugs free of charge to people who cannot afford them or whose insurance will not cover their use. The request for treatment must come from a physician, so these plans are often underutilized. People who cannot afford treatment are going without what they need because they aren't aware that it could be supplied without cost. If more people knew of opportunities like this, they surely would take advantage of them.

Right now, there are a few central sites that people turn to for information or support:

• **CancerNet** is a free electronic gateway into NCI information via Internet and other commercial services. You can get PDQ information summaries through your own computer by sending an e-mail message to:

cancernet@icicc.nci.nih.gov
Enter the word *HELP* in the body of the mail message.
To receive the information in Spanish, insert the word *SPANISH*.

CancerNet will send you a return-mail message with a list of CancerNet ID numbers, much like CancerFax, to use in requesting information.

• **OncoLink** is a leading resource for cancer patients and a popular meeting place for sharing information and support. It was founded and moderated by an especially knowledgeable and responsible sysop (system operator), but he has moved on, a victim of cyberpolitics. OncoLink remains, getting 15,000 calls ("hits") a day from 130 countries on everything from requests for the recipe for red-pepper sucking candy (for treatment-related mouthsores) to requests for help with reluctant HMOs. OncoLink's World Wide Web site address is http://cancer.med.upenn.edu/

Tip: If you see Dr. Loren Buhle's name associated with a cancer forum, tune in.

DATABASE SEARCH SERVICES: LET THE EXPERTS DO IT FOR YOU

Over the past decade, a minuscule private computer database industry that concentrated originally on alternative treatments has vastly expanded to meet the demand for the enormously greater amount of information available. It's revolutionizing patients' relationship to health care professionals—and this is only the beginning.

If you don't have the time or ability to do methodical computer searches for yourself, professionals are available who can skillfully scan current world medical literature for reports of new treatments and other material specific to your case: foreign drugs, alternative treatments, and medical specialists. The cost of a search, up to several hundred dollars, could be a sound investment in your health, and tax-deductible at that; but what you get for your money can vary.

The more difficult and individual medical conditions are, the less likely there is to be a large body of information available. Ironically, that's when treatment choices must be most artful. In those situations, it's more important than ever to have a skilled and experienced oncologist who can incorporate the complexities into a personal treatment plan. A computer search might offer intelligent new options to consider because it can tap extensive files of possibly helpful information. Remember that the largest number of reports in the medical literature concentrate on treatment for *primary* occurrence of the commonest cancers. Rarer cancers have correspondingly less information available. And recurrences can be very individual, complicated by a person's poorer health after treatment or metastasis to distant sites and difficult organs.

If you decide to use a service, have the details of your case with you when you call. The person with whom you speak will take a detailed history. The more specific you can be about your disease and the treatment you've already had (if any), the more specifically recommendations can be tailored to you. They understand that you are seeking *treatment*, so they limit their reports to medication actually in use or in clinical trials, not laboratory or experimental evidence.

The services vary in the type and content of the information they provide. Some include information about alternative (nontoxic or supportive) therapies. Some evaluate the data they are sending, offering pros and cons without making recommendations (that's your responsibility). A few offer lists of specialized physicians or hospitals and other supplementary reference material.

Search services are private, for-profit businesses, many of which grew out of their founders' search for treatment information for their own disease. Some are well established, others very new to the field. A lot of the *basic* information you might be getting is available free in other ways, so try to get the most for your money. Ask your doctor whether he or she has computer access to PDQ. If you've called the CIS for selected clinical trials, also tell that to the search service to avoid duplication. Be sure to call CancerFax first for background information (then mention that you have that information already).

Among representative commercial data services are:

• *The Health Resource, Inc.*, is a very well regarded information service that researches cancer and other diseases, although cancer reports are usually considerably longer than others (and cost more) because of the greater amount of information available. An RN takes information about your medical condition and any special needs or interests you want researched in depth. The report you get is very thorough, annotated and highlighted where the researcher wants to draw your attention to a particularly relevant study or conclusion. The Health Resource includes a listing, by state, of specialists in the treatment of your type of disease and a survey of alternative or holistic practices that are associated with your type of disease. Call 501-329-5272.

• *CAN HELP*, established a generation ago by Patrick McGrady, a health writer, may be the longest-running search service devoted to cancer. CAN HELP specializes in alternative and holistic treatment literature more than some other services, and Mr. McGrady's vast experience is helpful. Call 360-437-2291.

• *Schine On-line Services* offers several levels of information, from reports drawn from PDQ to specialized research requests. They also search Embase, a European database of drug-based clinical trials. Schine will provide you with a list of medical libraries in your region. (Have the zip codes of areas around your own location handy.) The information you receive is an *abstract*, a summary of the information a paper or report contains, not the item itself. You may want to look up the entire report or to use the bibliography that ends it for additional information. Call 800-FIND-CURE or 401-751-3320.

Making Your Search

Call several services and interview them.   Ask about follow-up questions, updating, recommendations, and costs. Keep notes of what you'll get for your money so you can make comparisons.

State exactly what it is you want to know.   Whether you seek basic information or treatment suggestions for a complicated medical problem, the more clearly you can identify what you want to know, the more useful will be what you get back in response. Callers to search services are more savvy than they were years ago, better informed about their own cases. Investing your time before you call will mean that you get a better, more tightly focused report back.

After you use a service, give them some feedback.   Call back and tell them how useful the information was (or wasn't). A few services, aware that knowledge in the patient community has expanded, offer a money-back guarantee: If you already have the information they provide, they will refund the cost of their investigation. Fair enough.

Other Information Sources

So many commercial interests are rushing to meet the demand for information that it's impossible to make any general statement about the quality of what's being produced. As a guideline, the more unspecialized the source of information, the more likely it is to contain entry-level information for the medical consumer. So, for example, the health videotapes sold in many super-drugstores are supportive without being very informative. And how much useful information can you get from a five-minute recording from a 900-number telephone medical information service? If you are already reading this book, you are beyond the need for that information.

MAKING TREATMENT CHOICES

The time will come to make decisions. All that information, all that paper, all that *work*—it's for this. It can be very hard to make treatment decisions because they are so important, and they can seem (or be) irreversible.

Whatever the nature of the decision you have to make, and always assuming the participation of your doctor(s), you can move toward making choices by carefully evaluating the content of the material you saved because it had some bearing on your situation.

As you read, ask the same questions of each document so you're sure of what it's telling you. Take careful, organized notes, then compare them point for point:

What are the treatment goals?
What is the treatment process?
What are the risks and benefits?

Comparing Treatment Goals

Are the goals of different treatments the same? Or are there different expectations from different regimens? How wide is the spread among them? If one goal of treatment is cure (resuming life with no sign of disease), what is known about secondary cancers must be taken into account so later-developing toxicities are minimized. When cure is not a likely outcome but prolonging life is, chronic or long-term toxicities are undesirable because they diminish quality of life.

Are the results of one treatment thought to be better in any way than any another? Is the long-term survival or disease-free interval longer with one treatment than another?

Comparing Treatment Processs

Do the regimens differ only in their means to the same ends? Is the choice simply different drug combinations? If so, consider immediate and long-term side effects of drugs, as well as possible complications.

Do the regimens differ dramatically—a no-treatment regimen versus a bone-marrow transplant, or surgery versus no surgery? What is required of you physically can affect how you recover and how you feel about treatment and should be factored into your evaluation.

Do the long-term effects of treatments differ? short-term effects? Some treatments have permanent effects that may narrow your future options, so their benefits and effects must be carefully weighed.

Comparing Risks and Benefits of Treatment

How likely are you to benefit from a treatment protocol? Recognizing that the best regimen will not work in all patients, how likely are you to match the "fit" of people who benefit?

Do you know the risks of one treatment over another? Can you equate them with the difference in treatment outcome? Some treatments for prostate cancer can put a patient at risk for impotence and incontinence. There are other treatments that are not "standard." Are they equally effective? Are their outcomes the same?

Is a treatment with greater toxicity or risk worth taking? In some cases, greater toxicity may lead to greater benefit, but toxicities may kill—even if the cancer is cured. Decision making must be grounded in your own ability to physically tolerate aggressive treatment.

When you choose a treatment, you set out in a direction. It is not necessarily irrevocable nor does it mean that further choices (or modifications) will not be prudent. The road chosen may have forks. When you come to one, evaluate the new conditions in the same deliberate way and select the direction in which you'll proceed. It's still going forward.

HOW TO GET INTO A CLINICAL TRIAL

If a clinical trial is your treatment choice, it can be easy to get into— *if* you fit the protocol and *if* it is open for enrollment.

The information you have about the trial probably comes from PDQ, which has an abbreviated list of entry criteria. *You cannot enroll yourself in a clinical trial* (except in rare circumstances). If you are interested in a particular trial, discuss it with your physician, who must evaluate your medical condition in terms of the trial criteria and make the arrangements for your enrollment, although you may have made the initial inquiries. Many oncologists are members of institutional or regional oncology groups that take part in clinical trials.

Trials, especially Phase III trials of longer duration and greater patient numbers, may have many sites. If there is one near you, your participation is more feasible. If you are being treated at a Clinical Cooperative Group or Community Clinical Oncology Program (see Chapter 4), you are more likely to have easy access to clinical trials, because they are NCI-supported research institutions.

The phenomenon of informed patients seeking clinical-trial information on their own, determining for themselves whether to join a trial, is quite new. Just a few years ago, the information about trials themselves was only available through physicians. It is not beyond the realm of imagination to speculate that the system is going to continue to change as the amount of information expands and as patients' rights becomes more of an issue. Much about the trial process should change also. (See Chapter 5.) The only hope that it will is through an empowered, aware patient community.

HOW TO READ SCIENTIFIC PAPERS

Services that provide information usually include a literature search consisting of abstracts (summaries) of reports drawn from medical journals. If you find an abstract with particular relevance to your case, you might want to read the complete paper, but you might feel intimidated by the content as well as the flat, formulaic style of scientific writing. (You'll rarely find any evidence of personality or journalistic art in scientific writing; impersonality is considered a virtue.) Nevertheless, you can develop a technique for reading a scientific paper so you get the information you need.

Basically, there are two types of papers: experimental results and literature reviews. Reviews are surveys of all the articles on a topic: straightforward background information or an overview of different opinions on a single subject. They are easily read with no special preparation. Experimental papers are less accessible, but you'll find them easier to read when you have the knack of doing it. *Read selectively.* You don't have to read every word nor every section to get what you need out of a paper.

Papers have distinct parts:

- *Title:* A long statement that tells you exactly what the paper is about. If you have trouble understanding the title, say it aloud, word by word, until you do understand. Then put it into your own words—saying, This paper is about (whatever)—so the subject is clear to you before you move on to the next part.

- *Author(s):* Listed in order of descending involvement or seniority. The authors' academic affiliations are listed as a footnote somewhere in the paper, and you are told with whom to correspond if necessary. You should get to know the names of significant researchers in your area of interest so you recognize them.

- *Abstract:* A concise overview of the paper, sometimes entitled Background. Usually only one paragraph of varying length, it is commonly set in italic or boldface type to set it apart from the paper itself. The abstract restates the problem, tells why the experiment was undertaken, how it was done, and the results it produced. It ends with the authors' conclusions and some indication of the direction of future research. After the title, the abstract is your next most useful summary of the paper. Read the first and last few sentences; skip the technical details until you have a good grasp of the content.

- *Introduction:* Background information telling you what the problem is that makes it necessary to do the research experiment. It is valuable reading. The authors explain state-of-the-art concepts of the aspect of the problem with which their work is concerned; they define the issues and offer evidence that the research they are doing can answer a specific question. Go slowly through this, and don't get bogged down in numbers or statistics. Read for information.

- *Materials and methods sections:* The fine print of a scientific paper. All the specifics are in this section: which patients or populations participated; what type of study it was; drugs that were used (if any), who supplied them, and how they were administered; and how the statistical analysis of the results was done. You can probably go through this quickly, unless you have reason to analyze the trial methods.

If you do wish to analyze the trial methods, *take notes as you read* so that differences between things become apparent. For instance, you might have two different patient groups with breast cancer, pre- and post-menopausal women. If the experiment involves high- and low-dose treatment, it could get confusing. Making a diagram like the following could help sort out information:

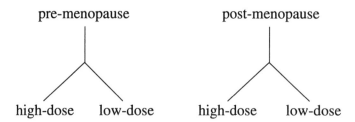

Then break down the grouping further, if necessary, or make notes next to each set. Diagramming treatment protocols makes them much easier to follow.

* *Results:* Observations of what happened over the course of the experiment. There can be a lot of statistics in this section. Ignore them. In a peer-reviewed journal, experts assess the statistics for credibility. The paper wouldn't be published if they were questionable.

* *Discussion:* The authors' thoughts about the meaning of the experiment and how the results contribute to understanding or treating the disease. The Discussion is "must" reading. It may seem difficult, but read slowly, aloud when necessary. Highlight only key phrases and key sentences. (A sure sign that you are not identifying the key concepts is that too much is underlined.) Make notes of the key points so you don't have to keep rereading the paper if you need to refer back to it later.

This section contains the majority of numbered references (enclosed in parentheses) to specific papers cited in the References. Science progresses by having each person's contributions added to the existing body of knowledge, so researchers' citations provide a foundation for their own paper.

* *References:* A list of articles referred to in the paper.

4

ON THE CUTTING EDGE

What You Should Know about Experimental Drugs

Today's cutting-edge experimental drug may well be the standard treatment of tomorrow. But the cutting edge is an uncomfortable place to be: It's sharp and it's very thin; there's no margin for error. You can get hurt on the cutting edge.

With cancer, though, we don't always have the luxury of options. Sometimes we have to take the risk of an experimental drug for a chance of its benefit. So it's important to understand what that risk really is—or what the promise is in a "promising" treatment.

As the public grows more experienced about cancer treatment and becomes much more sophisticated consumers of global medical news and breakthroughs, there is a noticeable increase in demand for drugs earlier in their development process. It is more important than ever that you know how to get through and around our own relatively unresponsive and rigid system, know how to get information, and understand the impact of public pressure on the development and timely availability of new therapies. You must get to know how the system works and why it is the way it is.

JULIE'S CASE

Julie's ovarian cancer was discovered six months after the birth of her baby. That baby, now five years old, and his older sister, have never been part of a normal family because, in normal families, Mommy doesn't have cancer.

Julie spends hours on the telephone, researching treatments or speaking with other patients about any developments they've heard of, anything new that might work. Inevitably, those telephone conversations are interrupted by her children demanding attention. They seem to hate the phone; it's part of the disease that keeps their mother from them.

Julie feels guilty that childhood has been stolen from her daughter and son by her illness. She anguishes over the effect on the children of living with worry—about disease, about side effects of drugs that treat disease, about fear of new disease. At the same time, she drives the children to excel. Just below the surface of her concern, one feels her anxiety: They may have to learn to manage without me. "I want my children to know me," she says. "I don't want to die. But if I'm going to, I want them to know that I did everything I could to live."

At first, Julie followed her oncologist's recommended treatment. She had the conventional two-drug regimen through a port in her abdomen that delivered the chemicals directly to the tumor. Port implantation was still a new procedure. Plagued by problems, it clogged after six months and had to be removed. With six more months of intravenous treatment, the CA 125 ovarian cancer tumor marker fell into the normal range, a hopeful sign that chemotherapy was shrinking the tumor. The oncologist said there was no need for another second-look surgery: "If it comes back, we'll know soon enough."

One year later, the CA 125 was rising, and Julie was back in treatment. By this time, however, she had become aware of the burdensome problems facing cancer patients: insurance reimbursement, restrictions on access to treatment, politics. She wanted to become involved in cancer issues. In *Coping*, a magazine for cancer patients, she found a resource list that included CAN ACT, the sole advocacy organization concerned with the most crucial issue for people in treatment: the availability of new therapies. Her husband became a dedicated member of the Board and a cancer activist.

Meanwhile, Julie's treatment was not going well. Her slender body grew thin, then bony, with the onslaught of drugs. She had been chemotherapy-bald for so long that, when her hair grew back, she had new friends who did not even know she was blonde. When her tumor became resistant to the standard treatment drugs, she was eligible for treatment with Taxol®, the cutting-edge drug. But she had to stop after only a few months because of its rigorous side effects. And the cancer was advancing.

When Julie heard of a French treatment protocol that sounded promising, she was quickly on the phone to Paris. The French doctor, who spoke excellent English (a relief), sent her a copy of the protocol, which she brought to her oncologist with trepidation. It involved the use of already-approved drugs in an off-label use, so he would not have to go through the Food and Drug Administration (FDA) or the hospital Board for approval. Julie thinks that if the protocol had employed new drugs or had been more unorthodox, the doctor would have rejected it because of the bureaucratic problems and legal exposure.

"Doctors should have the right to be creative. Businesses want creative accountants: why shouldn't patients have creative doctors?" she asks.

The protocol seemed to work, but it made her too sick. She had to stop. What to do next? "The doctor gave me his sad face and said 'We just wait.' I said, 'That means that Julie just rots, right?'" Her voice is exasperated even as she relates past events, "But, it pays to be persistent."

One day, she read an article in *Scientific American* about CAI, a potential treatment for ovarian and colon cancers, still in the early stages of development. The young National Cancer Institute (NCI) researcher who led the development team hoped that it would detect and kill very small early cancers, which are otherwise hard to find just at the stage when they are most treatable.

The cancer business is surprisingly democratic: Almost any cancer researcher is available to patients who are persistent enough. Julie called the principal investigator of CAI, but she was disappointed to learn that it was not ready for human trials.

By this time, she knew enough to be both persistent and pragmatic. She asked the researcher, a bright young woman about her own age, whether she could suggest anything else, whether anyone at the NCI was working on something new that would be suitable for her to try. Anything!

"Yes, perhaps photodynamic therapy," the doctor said. It sounds like a treatment imagined by a science-fiction writer, but it's real. Patients with certain susceptible cancers are injected with a substance that is particularly attracted to cancer cells. The substance lies dormant until a special laser is beamed directly on organs that contain it (a surgical procedure), causing microscopic "explosions" that kill the cancer cells.

"I felt like a vampire," she laughs. The procedure required her to reside away from light at NCI for more than a month, half of it in intensive care, followed by two more months in darkness at home.

"You always have to be your own advocate. No matter how dedicated, valiant, and interested your doctor is, he has a million other patients. My oncologist may like and respect me, but my life isn't valuable to him. I'm just a patient."

A troubled expression crosses her face. "Do doctors get tired of fighting paperwork? A lot of patients like me end up managing their own case. People look for something: Did *something* escape his attention? I found out about CAI before he did. He hears about stuff *that already has a track record*, from medical meetings and journals. We can't always wait until something has a track record. Somebody's got to get it first."

The effects of the photodynamic therapy lasted only a year. But by then CAI was ready for human trials, and Julie was ready for CAI.

WHERE NEW TREATMENTS COME FROM

New therapy drugs are developed collaboratively by three different institutions whose goals and constituents allow—or force—them to cooperate for the benefit of humankind. They are the NCI and the FDA, both branches of the U.S. Department of Health and Human Services, and, from the private sector, the pharmaceutical industry (including biotechnology). Their interests overlap and compete. Lines of responsibility are sometimes blurred, and suspicion of each other is rife. Yet new anticancer drugs emerge from the process and the public is the beneficiary.

Why You Should Understand the Drug Development Process

Treatment is the greatest concern of people with cancer, but only a limited number of effective drugs are available. Until they are diagnosed with the disease, most people don't understand how they are affected by the central issues about cancer:

Why there aren't more cancer drugs.   Cancer drug development is a slow process that always involves the FDA, usually the NCI, and a secretive private industry as well. Conflicting interests and strategic priorities can take precedence over the interests of patients.

Why some drugs are not available to your doctor for treatment use.   As you research new treatments, you may find that compounds mentioned are unavailable even when ample evidence of effectiveness exists. Regulatory barriers can keep them for years from where they will do the most good.

How to get around restrictions and barriers to new therapies.   If you want to obtain a drug that is still in development, you need to know how to work *with* the regulations in order to know how to work *around* them.

Why there isn't an effective voice for the rights and interests of people with cancer.   There is too little cancer advocacy. Pressure from the cancer community, judiciously applied, could encourage the development and approval of more treatments. Too many people think that raising money for research is all they can do. But unless research translates into treatment, it cannot help anyone but laboratory researchers.

The Role of the NCI

As the nation's largest single sponsor of research in cancer drugs, with nearly 200 compounds in clinical trials and even more in preclinical stages of development, NCI influences much more research than it conducts directly in its own extensive laboratory-hospital complex in Bethesda, Maryland. The agency contracts out research to academic institutions and has complex development ventures with private industry because it has neither the financial resources nor the authorization to market the drugs its researchers devise.

NCI controls a network of research and treatment-delivery centers in order to apply scientific advances to medical treatment. Patients in these institutions have a greater-than-average chance of being asked to participate in a clinical trial. Several NCI-designated cancer centers (and others) have allied to form a coalition that, it is hoped, will influence the standards of care in the somewhat uncertain future. The National Comprehensive Cancer Network, many of whose member institutions already represent state-of-the-art treatment, hopes to offset the loss of patients by offering specialized services to managed care providers.

- *Comprehensive Cancer Centers* or *Clinical Cancer Centers* (CCCs) are more than fifty NCI-designated treatment institutions sprinkled around the country. Clinical Centers emphasize basic scientific research as well as medical care, whereas Comprehensive Centers provide a more multidisciplinary approach to patient care. Both participate in research studies, which means that they have a higher proportion of clinical trials easily available to patients. Many large, well-known CCCs have extensive connections with community hospitals, making progressive research and treatment facilities available in less centralized areas.
- *Community Clinical Oncology Programs* (CCOPs, pronounced "C-cops") enable community-based, local oncologists to participate in clinical trials sponsored by the CCOGs or CCCs. Each CCOP is expected to provide a certain number of patients for trials each year. Some CCOPs concentrate on such specializations as problems of minority populations or pediatric cancers.
- *Clinical Cooperative Groups* (CCOGs, pronounced "C-cogs"), are investigators who work on the same research projects (protocols) cooperatively, pooling data and sharing administration. These can be regional (e.g., SWOG—Southwest Oncology Group; ECOG—Eastern Clinical Oncology Group), or they can be based on similar research focus (e.g., GOG—Gynecological Oncology Group; NSABP—National Surgical Adjuvant Breast Project; POG—Pediatric Oncology Group).

The Role of the FDA

The FDA shares responsibility for drug development through its mandate from Congress to protect the public from harmful food or drugs. It is a powerful partner in the drug development process because, over the years a drug is in clinical trials, *it alone is responsible for protecting human subjects of research.* FDA works with the drugs' sponsors to design and conduct trials that will satisfy its stringent requirements for proof of safety and effectiveness.

When bureaucratic government agencies have broad policy mandates, there are inevitably conflicts of interest in interpreting the *intent* of policies and the areas of authority. FDA has a cautious, safety-driven interpretation of its obligation to protect the public that prevents people with life-threatening illness from having new, possibly lifesaving drugs in timely fashion. Occasionally, NCI's *medical* priorities conflict with FDA's view of its *regulatory* responsibilities when a drug's entire effects are incompletely understood or when they present some risk.

In the past decade, AIDS activism was directed against conservative, risk-averse policies at both agencies. Since then, political forces targeted at the rigid procedures of the FDA and NCI have brought about radical change, and cancer drug development has benefited from more sensible, flexible policies and more humane priorities.

The Role of the Pharmaceutical Industry

The third important contributor to the development of new treatment drugs is the hugely successful, zealously private pharmaceutical industry. Although pharmaceuticals were formerly known as "ethical drugs," there are many who question the present scruples of this vital industry. Among the important public-policy questions we must ponder:

What are industry's priorities? In deciding which drugs to produce, does industry place profitability over need? Developing new drugs is a high-cost, high-risk venture. Companies might decide to produce a "copycat" drug to share a large, profitable market rather than invest in a drug for a disease that strikes only a small number of people.

What is the public responsibility of private industry? Some "breakthrough" drugs have contributed to the health and quality of life of people with cancer, but at a cost that is prohibitive for many. In some other countries, drugs cost less because government regulation controls profit. Are pricing policies fair to patients? Should private companies *have* to be fair?

How much profit is appropriate and necessary to encourage industry to produce drugs? If price regulation discouraged drug companies from producing profitable drugs, they might stop producing *un*profitable drugs. Many cancer drugs are not profitable, considering the cost of their development. Where would new cancer drugs come from if not from drug companies? As a society, we must consider how to balance competing interests.

"MAGIC BULLETS" TO "SMART DRUGS": WHY WE NEED TARGETED TREATMENT

Almost a century ago, the German bacteriologist Paul Ehrlich, who discovered the first effective treatment for syphilis and who also advanced cancer research, described treatments as "magic bullets" that would seek their own targets. Unfortunately, the weapons of the war on cancer are still very destructive, attacking cells without distinguishing between enemies and innocent bystanders.

The newest research directions focus on specific molecules, components, or processes of cancer cells. These "smart drugs" (it is hoped) will find their designated targets without the adverse effects of most chemotherapy drugs on normal healthy tissue.

All systemic treatments either kill malignant cells or interfere with tumor formation by preventing cancer cells from dividing and replicating. But systemic treatments within the body can have nonspecific toxic effects. The goal of cancer treatment has always been to gain the most specific effect while causing the fewest complications and side effects, because:

- *Drugs kill normal, healthy cells.* The basic problem of discovering lethal drugs that will not cause equal harm to normal cells has still not been solved. This is possibly because malignant cells come from cells that were originally normal and differ from them only slightly at first. When you lose your hair in chemotherapy, you have visible evidence of the nonspecific effects of toxic drugs.

- *The amount of time drugs can be used is limited.* The damaging effects of drugs limit the time that is acceptable or even possible for patients to have aggressive chemotherapy. Virtually all of the drugs deplete the immune system dangerously. Some place serious strain on the heart. Others are seriously debilitating and cause a fatigue problem. If some of those consequences could be eliminated or minimized, it might be possible to control cancers with prolonged chemotherapy. Perhaps someone could spend a lifetime "in remission"—the cancer not cured, but controlled. The outlook for people with diabetes, hemophilia, hypertension, and many other illnesses has been revolutionized by the development of lifelong, disease-controlling treatments. Perhaps someday, everyone with cancer will be that fortunate.

HOW NEW DRUGS ARE DISCOVERED

Some of the earliest chemotherapy drugs developed are still among the most widely used. It takes a long time to produce, let alone perfect, a new treatment for cancer and then explore its full potential. Every possible treatment for cancer goes through the same process of research, development, and approval. It is lengthy and, in many ways, unending. Once a drug is approved, it may seem to remain in clinical trials forever. However, combinations with newer agents are constantly being developed, and dosages and schedules refined.

Basic Science, Basic Scientists

The idea that a drug might be useful against cancer can come about in different ways:

- *By chance observation.* Scientists are trained observers of natural occurrences. When something unexpected happens, they want to understand why.

Platinum as a chemotherapy drug was discovered in 1965 as a result of a study of the effects of electric current on cell division in the common intestinal bacterium *E. coli*. Bacteria placed in special electric chambers were prevented from dividing to produce new bacteria only when platinum electrodes were used in place of electrodes made of more common metals. The researchers, curious about the unforeseen deadly effect on the cells, altered the experimental conditions one by one until they identified the cause: platinum. Although the original purpose of the study was different, researchers devoted years to experimenting with platinum. A platinum-based drug finally entered clinical trials in 1972. Since then, its two forms, cis-platinum and carbo-platinum, have contributed uniquely to the treatment of many cancers.

- *By logical deduction.* Some anticancer drugs are discovered because of the idea that something *should* be useful against cancer cells because of its known biochemical or other properties.

In 1944, very little was known about the structure or function of DNA, our genetic material. But two researchers with an idea that it should be possible to prevent the genetic replication of malignant cells spent years isolating potential agents to accomplish that goal. By 1953, they had a substance that effectively treated children with acute lymphocytic leukemia (ALL). Until then, the average child survived the disease only a few months. Today, a child diagnosed with ALL has an 80 percent chance of cure. For their pioneering work, the two researchers won the Nobel Prize (for Physiology or Medicine) in 1988.

- *By planned opportunity.* Every year, all over the world, thousands of substances are discovered to have some activity against cancer. In order to isolate the most promising candidates for further study, the NCI has a high-technology, high-volume strategy: the Preclinical Antitumor Drug Discovery Screen, available to all individuals and institutions, public and private. A dozen types of human cancer-cell cultures are used in computer-controlled measurement of antitumor activity. About 10,000 compounds are tested annually, in duplicate, at five different strengths, in different cell lines of each of the cell types. The result is: 12 million tests, or approximately 50,000 tests *daily.*

Limitations on Medical Development

Nonetheless, there are many frustrating limitations on the advances we may expect.

- *Technical limitations.* Scientists do not have ready-made solutions for all problems, and some are maddeningly elusive. Breast cancer research, for example, has been thwarted by the difficulty of growing common breast cancer cells in vitro. Whatever is different about breast cancer that makes it unusually difficult to grow in the laboratory is not yet understood. Researchers must overcome technical problems before they can solve the more subtle biological ones.

- *Goal limitations.* Scientists do not seem driven to solve the riddle of cancer in the same way, say, as many do of AIDS. As a result, a certain professional detachment has developed about cancer—a lack of urgency. With the recent rise of breast cancer activism, research money poured into labs—and scientists followed. It's a simple concept.

- *Cost limitations.* With fewer dollars available for research, diseases are competing for attention because attention attracts funding. The politicization of disease is a troubling development. People with different cancers shouldn't compete with each other for research in *their* type of disease because the solution for one type may come from a breakthrough in another type.

PRECLINICAL TESTING: CAN THIS STUFF BE USED AGAINST CANCER?

In Vitro

The earliest stages of research are conducted *in vitro* (in glass), the ubiquitous hardware of laboratories. Cultures of bacteria, viruses, or cancer cells are utilized as research material, but no higher animals are involved.

Evidence that a substance has *some sort of desirable effect against tumor cells* alone determines whether it goes any further in preclinical research. Studies of *toxicology* (the negative side effects an agent might have) are neither possible nor necessary this early in the process, because the effects are likely to be different in mammals. Designing drugs in the laboratory is theoretical. Whether a new drug is developed by a computerized drug screen or by a researcher with an inspiration, the end product must still be tested in living subjects.

In Vivo

When a substance is identified in vitro to have activity against cancer cells, research moves on to *in vivo* (in life) studies: testing in animals. The test substance, in varying doses or for varying periods of time, is administered to a group of specially bred rats or mice that predictably develop a variety of specific cancers. The effects are meticulously followed. A second, matched group of laboratory animals is used as a *control* group. Instead of the test substance, they are treated with an inert or biologically inactive substance.

Any difference in the development of cancer—its size or the course of its progression—or the length of time of survival of the treated group indicates that the substance may be useful against cancer and warrants further study. Tumor response alone—whether it shrinks or disappears as a result of exposure to the new compound—is the sole initial interest. As research progresses, *dose-modification studies* are begun to identify a dose that is both effective *and* safe—one that will kill the active cancer without killing the animal (or, later, the human patient).

At the same time, the original substance may be undergoing studies to identify and isolate the active ingredients. When that has been accomplished, the compound can be made up in quantity and in a uniform quality. Finally, it will be turned into pills, injectable liquid, or another "delivery system" (perhaps a skin patch) so that it can be easily administered to research animals or human subjects. Few substances are effective or safe enough to survive preclinical testing: Of a possible 5,000 tested, only five will enter clinical trials.

CLINICAL TESTING: CAN THIS STUFF BE USED IN PEOPLE WITH CANCER?

In research in general, many new compounds are tested in healthy people or in volunteers with less-threatening medical conditions. However, in cancer research, *the subjects are always cancer patients* because:

- Chemotherapy treatments work by interfering with two vital natural processes: (1) *metabolism,* the sum of all the chemical processes that allow us to live and grow, and (2) *cell division*, the process that is necessary for normal growth and repair. It would be unthinkable to interfere with either in normally healthy people.

• Many compounds have powerful oncogenic, teratogenic, or mutagenic cumulative or side effects.

Oncogenic effects lead to the development of other cancers, often years after the primary treatment. Increasingly, long-term survivors of childhood and other cancers face late-developing secondary cancers caused by toxic chemotherapy drugs.

Teratogenic effects of chemotherapy (and other) drugs damage developing fetuses (without causing hereditary changes in the mother's DNA). The disastrous events associated with the sleep-inducing medication thalidomide provided a graphic lesson in the need for extreme caution when medicating during pregnancy. For that reason, pregnant women cannot have chemotherapy, nor can they participate in most clinical trials.

Mutagenic effects (mutations) are changes in an individual's genetic material, changes that can start the chain of cellular events that lead to cancer. Radiation of many kinds is known to cause the kind of chromosomal damage that is inherited.

There is one advantage to testing new drugs in people who already have the disease: At the same time that researchers are learning about possible toxicities, they are offering patients the possibility of therapeutic benefit.

PHASE I CLINICAL TRIALS: HOW SAFE?

Phase I clinical trials are toe-in-the-water tests: cautious, progressive studies. They seek answers to questions of safety:

• How much of the substance is it safe to take?
• How is the drug absorbed?

Notice that neither of those questions asks how *effective* the drug is against cancer. While "therapeutic intent" is always present, and, indeed, a compound would not be tested had it not already demonstrated anticancer activity in preclinical studies, Phase I trials are not *primarily* measurements of effectiveness against cancer—they are *safety* studies.

What Phase I Trials Accomplish

Phase I trials are dose-escalation studies.   Dose escalation, as you might guess, is like a staircase on which each step up represents an increase in quantity. Researchers devise tests that will show whether there are any toxic effects with increasing time or increasing dose and whether the effects are reversible.

Data from laboratory animal studies is used to establish the amount with the least toxic effects or the level at which the effects are reversible. The first group of patients, usually three to six, starts at the lowest dose level. If the substance proves safe and well tolerated after allowing enough time for delayed side effects to develop, a second group starts the test with a higher dose, and so on until the "maximally tolerated dose" (MTD) is reached, just a step down from "unacceptably toxic" side effects.

A safe starting dose in people must be established because safety testing in animals, even in large mammals like the dogs frequently used in research, does not necessarily translate exactly to human responses. Many Phase I drugs that show some effect against cancer never reach Phase II testing because they have destructive side effects even at very low levels. Investigators are particularly careful about organ-specific toxicities, such as heart or lung problems that might develop, because they are not always predictable.

Phase I trials are studies of the pharmacokinetics of drugs.   Scientists study how a drug is absorbed, where it ends up in the body, how it got there, how long a substance is retained in the blood or organs, and how (and how quickly) it is eliminated.

WHAT PHASE I TRIALS ARE NOT
- *They are not blinded.* Everyone knows which drug he or she is taking and so do the researchers.
- *They are not randomized.* Everyone who participates is assigned to take the known drug at known dose levels.
- *They are not comparison trials.* All participants are treated with the same new substance.

What You Should Know If You Are Thinking about Joining a Phase I Trial

If you are considering participating in the clinical testing of a Phase I drug, there are facts you should have before you begin.

Know how close to the MTD you might be and on which step you are starting.   You might want to start at a higher dose or a lower dose, depending on what you can find out about the clinical experience already accumulated. Some of this is negotiable, especially when you get to know the investigators.

Know the physical signs that will indicate that toxicities are developing.   Your health will be carefully monitored by trial personnel, but you should be monitoring yourself, too. We all respond somewhat unpredictably to different drugs, so the effects you experience might vary from what is expected. Although your doctor might be reluctant to discuss the toxicities for fear of evoking a "placebo response" (physical symptoms that come only from the belief that you will have them), be persistent. And telephone with questions as they arise.

Know your own disease and its standard treatment.   Patients who enroll in Phase I trials must have a malignancy that can be confirmed by physical tests or scans and that is not responsive to conventional treatments. Because there are significant risks in the use of therapies that are still in development, it is sensible to *exhaust all the standard treatment possibilities first*. To be accepted, you are usually required to have good kidney and liver function so that the drug can be eliminated from your system efficiently.

Phase I trials are brief.   Usually only a few weeks' duration, Phase I trials are generally conducted at single hospitals under the supervision of a single researcher and involve only a small number of patients. In that way, toxicities experienced by any patients are most easily recognized by the researcher when they develop in others. Trials involving several institutions and larger numbers of patients are only permitted when the risks are better understood and when the patient population that might benefit is more clearly identified.

There is one exception to the single-institution policy. Because of the relative rarity of cancer in children, the NCI recognizes that it is appropriate to involve several institutions in a single Phase I clinical trial for pediatric cancer.

For every hundred drugs that have the potential for becoming useful treatments through the clinical trial process, about seventy will complete Phase I. The other thirty will have shown problems of safety or other problems serious enough to eliminate them from further consideration.

Occasionally, a drug shelved for toxicity or lack of effectiveness will later be rescued from obscurity. Cis-platinum had just this history. After its fortuitous discovery in the mid-1960s, human clinical trials in the early 1970s demonstrated its potential. But severe gastrointestinal and kidney damage resulted from concentrations of the platinum, and it was nearly abandoned as a treatment. Not until several years later, when more effective antinausea medication had been developed and a regimen of hydration devised to clear the toxic metal from the kidneys more efficiently, was cis-platinum sufficiently tamed to be used therapeutically.

PHASE II CLINICAL TRIALS: HOW EFFECTIVE?

Phase II clinical trials look for answers to *therapeutic* questions:

- Which specific types of cancer might respond to the new drug?
- Which patients at what stages of disease are most likely to benefit?
- Which dose gives the most promising clinical response with the least toxicity, and how often should it be administered?

What Phase II Trials Accomplish

When a compound is identified that has some antitumor effect and a well-tolerated dose is established, researchers must learn how to use it effectively in people. Phase II clinical trials are tests designed to reveal more subtle information about the way the drug works. The trials are not randomized. Everyone is treated with the experimental compound, although dosage levels may vary.

Phase II trials show whether the drug retards the growth of tumors or is effective in some other way. In order to prevent too many unknown or variable factors from affecting the results, NCI encourages researchers to conduct *two* Phase II trials in each of the tumor types under study. By comparing the two sets of results, any unexpected or aberrant results will be evident.

They identify which tumors are sensitive to its effects and which are not. People in Phase II trials have various types of cancer. They are grouped by tumor type and matched as carefully as possible for age, gender, race, type and location of tumor, extent of disease, and many other clinical similarities.

They are used to study the best way to get the drug to the tumor (the "route of administration"). Oral, injectable, or infusible methods have many complexities. Although some drugs can be compounded in more than one form, for trial purposes, the most benign or expedient one is identified early.

What You Should Know If You Are Thinking of Joining a Phase II Trial

Phase II trials might have more than one stage. As Phase II trials progress and as knowledge of the specific action and target population for the new agent accrues, patients with less optimal conditions have an opportunity to participate in the trial. Eligibility requirements might be modified for the Phase II/Stage 2 participants so that you can benefit from what was learned in the first stage of the trial. A second stage offers investigators a broader, more representative patient base in which to study the new agent's usefulness; and patients have the benefit of treatment with a drug about which more is known.

There may be intermediate stages. More flexibility has been introduced into the rigid clinical-trial process in order to speed it up. Researchers work more closely to analyze data so that they may respond to promising results more quickly. NCI has inaugurated intermediate steps, Phase I–II and Phase II–III that combine elements of each phase, for certain promising drugs. (These intermediate steps are not FDA designations.) A little bit more—or a little less—might be known about a drug in a fast-tracked trial, but you have the advantage of knowing that there are reasons for special interest in these treatments.

Of the seventy potential new drugs left from the original hundred, another thirty-seven will be dropped for safety concerns during Phase II tests, or because they just don't work.

Thirty-three will complete Phase II testing and go on to Phase III.

PHASE III CLINICAL TRIALS: HOW GOOD?

Phase III clinical trials are conducted for *comparison* of a new drug with drugs that are already known to be effective. The trials offer the largest number of opportunities for your participation.

The most important questions that a Phase III trial asks are:

- Is the new agent an improvement over the standard drug (or experimental ones, if there is no "best treatment")?
- Does it work in a different way?
- Does it have fewer toxicities?

These later trials often ask broad, interesting questions that go beyond the simple and relatively straightforward one of whether a single drug is effective for a single cancer. A recent trial studied whether the same short-term, intensive, two-drug treatment program for breast cancer was more effective when given *before* or *after* two different types of surgery to remove the tumor, *either* radical mastectomy *or* lumpectomy. In that trial, women were grouped by age so that any differences in response would be clear. Participants were to be followed for five years before the results would be clear.

Another trial compared high-dose therapy with low doses of the same drug, with and without the addition of a biological-response modifier that is known to enhance the effect of one of the treatment drugs.

What You Should Know If You Are Thinking of Joining a Phase III Trial

Phase III trials are large-scale trials and may take several years. Phase III trials involve hundreds or even thousands of patients at many institutions. The more people involved, the more likely it is that the results will be broadly applicable—and provide reliable, convincing data. (But remember that *individual variability* is lost or overlooked in this format.) The NCI CCOGs are particularly active in involving patients in Phase III trials.

They are randomized, usually double-blinded, and carefully controlled. In an effort to maintain objectivity, participants are assigned to different groups (arms) of the trial as randomly as possible, usually by computer. A matched control group of participants does not receive the experimental compound, but neither doctors nor participants are aware of who is experimental and who is control.

They may involve more than one type of cancer. Phase III trials develop the information learned from Phase II studies, especially understanding which types of cancer respond to the new compound.

They are comparison studies. The experimental compound is compared to the standard regimen for one or more types of cancer.

Of approximately one hundred drugs that started the trial process, only twenty-five to thirty will be left after Phase III. Of that number, only twenty will one day be available as treatments.

5

TRICK OR TREATMENT

What No One Tells You about Clinical Trials

Less than 10 percent of patients enroll in clinical trials, regardless of the treatment opportunities they may offer. Why so few? Because the treatment you receive in a trial may not be the best treatment possible for you.

Joining clinical trials presents some patients with difficult choices—and doctors with complex ethical questions. If you are thinking about enrolling in a trial, you should carefully think through what's best for yourself. The issues are most serious for you. Doctors, researchers, and medical personnel can leave their work behind at five o'clock, but you still have cancer. Give yourself time to sort out the questions so that your own interests are always best served.

TREATMENT ISSUES

New Drugs versus Conventional Treatment

When is a new or untested drug better treatment for you than what is already available? According to the NCI, it is better:

1. When you have a cancer, such as liver cancer or pancreatic cancer, for which *no single-drug or combination-drug treatment is known to be effective.*

2. When the standard treatment is said to have *no impact on survival*. Even if chemotherapy leads to "objective regression" (measurable shrinkage of the tumor), statistics may show it has little or no ability to prolong life. Patients have a difficult choice to make in this situation because they cannot know how statistics apply to themselves. Statistics apply only to groups. Systemic therapy may help some people live longer, but not others. Or it may prolong the time of *disease-free* survival, even if the outcome is unchanged.

3. When, conversely, you have a type of cancer that usually responds to standard systemic therapy. NCI *encourages* patients to undergo experimental treatment, especially if they have had *no*, or only *minimal prior treatment* for their disease (*"For initial Phase II studies, we currently seek trials that restrict patient eligibility to the minimum extent of prior therapy consistent with ethical medical practice"*).*

Medical ethics dictate that patients should have the best treatment available, but the decision may be complicated for a patient who fits this profile. NCI justifies the guideline because people with minimal prior chemotherapy or radiotherapy have less compromised immune and organ systems, are perhaps healthier, and possibly have less-resistant tumors than people who have had extensive treatment.

For many types of cancer, *several different treatment* programs are known to bring about a response. You would be sensible to investigate or exhaust all possible therapeutic avenues before embarking on an early-stage trial in which there are many unknowns. Remember that the goals of the three phases of clinical trials are different. (See Chapter 4.)

Single-Agent versus Combination Chemotherapy

For a new drug to progress through clinical trials, two things must be proven:

- That it is doing what researchers *think* it does.
- That it *alone* is causing the observed effect.

*National Cancer Institute, Division of Cancer Treatment, *Investigator's Handbook* (Bethesda, MD: U.S. Department of Health and Human Services, October 1993).

Every drug is tested by itself in early-stage trials, although drugs are used *almost always* in combination. The challenge, if you are considering a clinical trial, is to compare the potential benefit of a *new drug used alone* (experimentally) against the effect of a *standard, multidrug treatment program.* How can you tell which would give you what you really want, or which is the better treatment? You don't want to risk having inferior treatment by participating in a trial, but what the better treatment is may not be obvious.

A half-century of experience with chemotherapy has shown that, for most cancers, a combination of drugs, used together or one after another in a series, is more effective treatment than one drug used alone. There are several reasons why this might be true:

- *Combined effects may be more potent* than the power of any one drug known individually to be effective.
- *Drugs work in different ways*, striking different targets within cells, reaching cells at different stages when they may be more susceptible to certain drugs, or possibly activating different components of our own immune systems.
- *Toxicities differ.* Although all drugs have side effects, some serious, they do not all have the same kind, nor do they show up at the same time. Spreading adverse effects around may mean a better quality of life for you.
- *Resistances may be delayed or avoided.* You might become resistant to one drug with prolonged treatment, but irregular exposure to several drugs may help prevent resistance from developing.

Measuring Response

When a drug in clinical trials is shown to be effective against cancer, what exactly does it mean to you? That it will cure your cancer? That you will live for two, ten, or twenty years? It doesn't mean anything of the sort.

- *Complete response* (CR, or complete remission) means that all evidence of disease disappears *for more than one month* and that your Karnofsky performance status (see p. 106) returns to a normal level.
- *Partial response* (PR, sometimes called positive response) means

that the tumor mass is reduced by the action of the drug to 50 percent or less of its original mass *for more than one month,* with no evidence of new disease.

Complex mathematical computations indicate the *likelihood* that you or anyone else will respond in the predicted way. It does not mean that you will—it's simply a statistical probability.

The very real and troubling problem for anyone considering enrolling in clinical trials is that the treatment you receive is likely to consist of one drug whose *standard for effectiveness is approximately one month's duration.*

Most trials are limited to a defined period of time or until results are obtained. Almost nothing that happens afterward is of the slightest concern to the researchers. However, you, for one, are *very* interested.

One standard ovarian cancer protocol consists of six periodic treatments of a two-drug regimen. There is a statistical probability of achieving remission by this protocol, but everyone (except maybe the patient) recognizes that the remission is, by definition, temporary. The regimen does not go on to suggest what (if anything) your doctor might do afterward, nor is there any indication of what effect the experimental treatment might have on follow-up treatment with standard therapies.

The cloud over clinical trials is the general feeling that they represent the "last ditch effort" for effective treatment, and that participating in a trial means you've run out of treatment (or even palliative) possibilities.

But you may have other treatment again following a trial, and you might benefit from it. Cancer treatment is a long-term project. Many treatments go on for several years, so don't expect that a two-month clinical trial is all you'll need. There's even a name for the treatment required after a drug has achieved significant beneficial effect. It's called *consolidation therapy*, and its goal is to consolidate the benefit of previous treatment.

Clinical Endpoints: Survival versus Surrogate

A clinical trial ends at the "endpoint"—when enough statistics have been collected to answer the question, "Is this drug effective against cancer?"

New drugs were generally approved if they fit a narrow standard for benefit:

- They *cured* tumors and brought about *survival.*
- They were *better* at treating cancer than other drugs already approved.

In 1991, ten scientists from NCI and FDA collaborated on a paper that suggested that broader standards should be set for new compounds—whether they promote the health, well-being, or prolonged survival of someone with disease. So that people with cancer would benefit from advances in medicine at the earliest possible time, they proposed for the first time that alternate, or surrogate, endpoints be used. (One surrogate marker familiar to almost everyone is the number of T cells in a person who is HIV-positive.)

Surrogate endpoints for cancer, ways to tell if drugs are having a desired effect, include:

> *Improved quality of life*, which includes a variety of elements: maintenance of normal weight, decreased dependence on medical support, ability to have outpatient treatment rather than hospital treatment, and such.
> *Longer disease-free time* before a recurrence.
> *Easing or disappearance of symptoms.*
> *Increased number or duration of complete responses.*

In the few years since 1991, the concept of surrogate endpoints for cancer has sensibly taken hold in research, but drug-approval policies still resist the idea of patient-benefit priorities. Once again, an involved, vocal representation by cancer patients in their own interests could improve the treatment picture without the spending of one additional dollar of research money.

How Label Indication Is Determined by Trials

You will find that many clinical trials are studies of drugs already in common use to treat other forms of cancer. That is how science is done, how it learns more about the uses of a drug. The conduct of clinical trials also has to do with how drugs are approved.

Clinical trials usually last only long enough to develop measurable response. A drug whose action is immediate and measurable will be considered effective even if the response lasts but a month. On the other hand, beneficial effect might not be noticed if the drug's effect is cumulative or delayed, and follow-up of people who leave clinical trials is inconsistent.

A drug's sponsor must prove that a new compound is beneficial, so it sensibly selects *the best demonstration of what is known at that time* about:

- The type of cancer that best shows the drug's effect.
- The length of treatment sufficient to get the best effect at a tolerated dose.
- How to get the drug into a person's system.

When a drug is approved by the FDA, those specifics become the "label indication." Doctors can use the new drug against other cancers, helping people with the disease while adding to knowledge of the other uses of the drug ("off-label" uses). Often, the best use or the most effective dose of a new therapy is discovered only after it is approved, perhaps for a different cancer.

Reliable reports of off-label uses of approved drugs fill medical literature. When physicians use drugs off-label, in a different indication or in combination with other drugs as based on evidence from experimental medical literature or their own experience, they may risk not being paid by third-party payers. *You* risk not receiving the best medical treatment or not having the treatment reimbursed or paid for by your insurer, *even when it is part of the most effective treatment regimen.*

When clinical trials proclaim a new drug effective, you can see that it is a rather qualified determination. Newer uses *might* eventually be added to the package insert—if the manufacturer wishes to go through the lengthy (and costly) procedure. Even so, there is a time lag during which more and more current information is accumulating. Conceivably, the label uses would never catch up to actual use.

The label indication is not a cookbook. It may not even reflect standard treatment for cancer, and it may not be the best treatment for cancer. The problem of label indications and off-label use is a problem that may only be resolved when we and our doctors prevail on the FDA to update its standard to reflect everyday medical practice.

CLINICAL TRIAL ISSUES

Entry Criteria: Can You Get In? Can You Get Out?

All trials have "inclusion criteria" and "exclusion criteria" that tell you clearly who is and isn't suitable for the trial.

Inclusion criteria tell you what *you must have* to get into the trial. They identify a group of patients with the greatest similarity to each other. People are classified by sex, age, and disease condition (type, stage, amount of previous treatment) into groups called "cohorts." (There can be several cohorts in a trial: pre- and post-menopausal women, for example.) Too much variation within the group would require subjective explanation and "confound" the results.

Although every researcher would like to have as many people recruited into his or her trial as possible, it often works out the other way: too few patients or too slow accrual. In general, when fewer people are available to participate in a trial, in the case of rare diseases, the inclusion criteria are more flexible.

Clinical trial results are data—numbers and statistics—not biographies or subjective impressions. Statistics sort out the effects of the drug from the effects of disease. Analysis of clinical trial data is as objective as possible.

Exclusion criteria tell you what conditions will *keep you out* of it. They are typically medical conditions that would be complicated or made worse by use of the experimental agent.

A history of cardiovascular problems and hypertension usually restricts your participation. Pregnancy is always contraindicated in a trial for a cancer drug, and many trials require women to use contraception; some require men to do the same. (It is in your own interest to cooperate.) Kidney diseases may prevent you from participating in a trial because the kidneys concentrate urine prior to excretion and may be damaged by quantities of a drug the urine contains.

Impaired reasoning and organic brain damage are always limitations that exclude participants because the ability to give informed consent is questionable.

Secondary cancers may be grounds for exclusion, but that varies with what is being tested. Most skin cancer patients who have been successfully treated are acceptable. But in many trials, especially longer ones, a person with prior melanoma will be excluded (except from a melanoma trial). This is because the long-term survival of melanoma patients is poor at present, and some trials require long-term follow-up for statistical credibility. Those trial designs coldly exclude patients who may not live until the end of the trial or confound the data by dying before the trial is completed.

Trials usually require that some period of time elapse since prior treatment so that drugs will not intermingle, a concern that protects *you* as well as the reliability of the research data.

Most trials specify that participants must have "measurable disease parameters"—tumor that is measurable either physically (perhaps a skin cancer) or with diagnostic probes such as CAT scans or X rays. Any change in the tumor resulting from treatment can, thus, be measured, quantified and described. In certain circumstances, the limitation of measurability will be bypassed. If a tumor, perhaps a bone metastasis or a brain lesion, cannot be measured physically or assessed in other objective ways, a clinical trial participant may be evaluated for response by the investigators (more than one, to ensure objectivity).

Performance Status

Every trial has "performance status" standards. There are several in common use, all of which measure your health and quality of life before and during your participation in research with an experimental substance, so that any changes that arise as side effects can be noted. Professionals evaluate you, but you are not usually told your status.

All performance status evaluations use a numerical or similar scale. Confusingly, some of them (ECOG, AJC) indicate deterioration by going from zero (normal activity) *up* to four (a bedridden patient or someone who needs hospitalization), while others logically go *down* (e.g., the Karnofsky scale: someone with no evidence of disease who does normal activities is rated 100 percent; a person requiring considerable assistance and frequent medical attention is rated 50 percent; a person rated below 10 percent has fatal processes under way).

Other measurements of blood values or organ function tell how well they are working under the added stress of chemotherapy or other intrusive treatment. Some of the common markers are:

- *Creatinine clearance:* Measures kidney function. Creatinine, a protein found in the blood, is excreted through the kidneys in urine. Lower creatinine levels indicate lower kidney function.
- *Bilirubin, transaminase (SGOT, SGPT), and alkaline phosphatase:* Measure liver function. Because the liver detoxifies dangerous substances, its ability to function normally is especially important. Elevated levels of the marker substances indicate lowered ability of the liver to clear toxic substances.
- *Blood counts—WBC (white cells); RBC (red cells); PLT (platelets); Hgb (hemoglobin), granulocytes, and lymphocytes:* Measure the amounts of components of your blood. White-cell depletion, called neutropenia or leukopenia, is a common side effect of many cytotoxic drugs. In most blood test values, lower numbers indicate higher toxicity, although an elevated white cell count can suggest other problems.

(Any good library has medical reference books for consumers that contain complete information about the tests, normal and abnormal values, and what they mean.)

CONSENT ISSUES

Informed Consent

It may be that the last time you gave your informed consent you found yourself with a spouse. When you give informed consent to participate in a clinical trial, you can be sure you'll be better prepared.

- *Informed consent* is a legal document stating that you choose of your own free will to be treated.

- It is a safeguard to prevent your being treated with anything against your will.
- It ensures (to the degree possible) that you understand that there are unknown risks in taking a new drug or having a new procedure and that there is no guarantee of benefits.

The shocking violations of medical-research ethics that have come to light make informed consent a matter of everyone's concern. The notorious Tuskegee Study of Untreated Syphilis in the Negro Male shows the potential for exploitation. For forty years, U.S. Public Health Service doctors monitored the progress of the disease known for centuries to lead inevitably, if not treated, to deterioration, insanity, and death. The doctors who ran the study enticed 430 black residents of rural Macon County, Alabama, to participate by offering free "treatment" for what was called colloquially "bad blood." Participants were not told that they had syphilis, nor that treatment consisted only of placebos and tests—for the real purpose of the study was to observe the natural, untreated course of the disease. Most of the patients died in pain and suffering.

Only in early 1972, when a government panel released a report, was the study officially discontinued. No evidence was found that the patients had given any kind of informed consent, and the panel concluded that the study was unjustified on both scientific and humanitarian grounds. Deplorably, more than ten years elapsed from the time an African-American epidemiologist sought an investigation of this shameful episode until he succeeded in having it shut down.

The Tuskegee story was disclosed at a time when the inhuman abuses of inmates of concentration camps in Europe and the Nuremberg Code, a formal statement of medical ethics that protects the rights of human research subjects, were still somewhat fresh in the minds of Americans. Guided by the Code, the Public Health Service (PHS) defined informed consent and made it a condition of PHS research funding. In time, a national commission was appointed to develop recommendations for the protection of human subjects of biomedical and behavioral research, which were later converted into the informed consent regulations now enforced by the FDA.

Now, decades later, the punctilious adherence to sometimes overly protective guidelines can appear to be excessive. Is it?

Troubling revelations of unethical radiation experiments conducted by the military in the years *after* World War II prove that people concealed knowledge of the events until the present. Soldiers were used in experimental studies but not informed of their "participation" nor of the risks to which they were subjected. Experiments included injecting eighteen men with radioactive plutonium to study its course through the body and exposing both humans and animals to unprotected close-up views of atomic blasts in order to study the resulting effects on eyes, which included damage to the retina.

Plainly, abusers do not announce their intentions. If you are going to volunteer for a clinical trial, you should be skeptical and vigilant. Most important, *have the confidence* to question those in authority.

Studies versus Clinical Trials

Could you unwittingly participate in a study without your informed consent? Possibly. Ninety percent of hospitals and institutions have "assurance agreements" that they will abide by rules and regulations that govern research in human subjects, including informed-consent provisions. Federal funding of research mandates such agreements; and because most institutions are the recipients in one way or another of government money, adherence is guaranteed.

A small percentage of research institutions do not have established agreements to comply with federal guidelines. It does not mean that they can abuse research subjects because there are local laws protecting people. But it does mean that you might be given a modified treatment regimen, dose, duration of treatment, or drug combination *without your knowledge or consent.*

Most researchers are reluctant to admit that there are studies that are not out-and-out clinical trials, but they exist. Ask your oncologist whether your proposed treatment is part of a study. If it is, it does not mean that it is worse or more dangerous than conventional treatment. It may even become conventional treatment if it proves superior. But you should be the one to decide whether you will participate in a study.

Who's Afraid of Informed Consent?

In our blame-riddled society, the giving and taking of informed consent has become charged with suspicion from the givers *and* the takers. The public may never feel sufficiently protected, and it cannot rely on the humanitarian values of researchers. In medical settings, more than any others, interests overlap but potential *conflicts* of interest exist.

Clinical trials involving human subjects is expensive, time-consuming, and labor-intensive. Funding for research is scarce and somewhat centralized. Consequently, only successful protocols are likely to garner funds (for the researcher). If patients quit the study or decline to participate, the reputation or validity of the study itself may suffer, and the investigator may find it difficult to garner support for subsequent work.

Surprisingly, it is the medical profession that is shy about facing informed consent squarely. It may be that they are more honest about the unknowns in medicine in an outright experimental setting than in the clinic.

Next time you have a procedure in or outside of a clinical trial that requires your written consent, notice when the form is handed you to sign. It probably will not be mailed to you to study *in advance*, nor will it be given to you while you wait for the appointment. More likely it will be handed to you after elaborate preparations for your procedure or treatment have been completed, just as it is ready to start. (And try reading the small print while everyone is waiting for you to *just sign!*)

What are doctors afraid of? That we will understand that there are risks in the procedure, that the doctors guarantee nothing, and that the tissue they take belongs to them? (In fact, there have been lawsuits about each of those points.)

We patients must accept responsibility for our share of risk. The working out of this lack of understanding has been through the judicial process, where patients have sought relief from perceived and real abuses. The medical side has responded by practicing "defensive medicine," following conservative practices that emphasize safety and avoidance of legal exposure, generally taking no "heroic measures," and treating according to academic guidelines. Certainly it does not include making the dramatic, possibly lifesaving therapeutic interventions for which American medicine has become deservedly famous—and that in many ways advanced its knowledge, practice, and expertise.

If you are taking a risk, make it an *educated* risk. With as much information as you can get, compare the risk with the possible benefit. Researchers are obliged to provide sufficient information to participants in a clear, understandable manner so they can consent to participating with the understanding that all the effects are not known.

It helps to speak frankly with your doctor, reassuring her or him that you know there are risks in the procedure or treatment and that you know you need it. Then ask which complications might occur and which are unlikely. Nevertheless, you cannot be sure that all or even sufficient information *is* being given to you. You do not even know how much information will make you *fully* informed. So how fully informed can you be? There is no absolute answer. You should satisfy yourself to the extent possible—and *keep asking questions.*

Signing the Consent Form

There is no single, universal, official informed consent document, although there are very specific NCI-required and optional elements for clinical trials. Each institution responsible for the conduct of a trial develops its own form, but all consent forms will tell you:

Your participation is voluntary and optional. You don't have to consent to anything. But if you want to participate in the trial, you must give formal, signed consent, and usually more often than once. Signed forms are mandatory for the clinical investigator and the drug's sponsor to have. If the guidelines for a trial change (as they frequently do), you must be informed again and sign a new document to show it. Any time you want to stop participating in the trial, you can just drop out—and stop consenting. The form also tells you that it is your right to do so.

Your involvement is confidential. It is a secret between you and your physician—and the insurance company, the sponsor, the FDA, and the NCI. (Some secret!) The research may end up published in a medical journal, but your name will not be attached to it, so it can never find its way into publication. There are many reasons to keep it that way, but chiefly because health insurance companies will generally not reimburse you for treatment administered in a clinical trial. (Unfortunately, they usually know.) The confidentiality works both ways, because the drug's sponsor is equally intent on keeping a proprietary rein on information.

What the research is about.   You are receiving a new medication and you should know what benefits might be expected (tumor shrinkage or nausea suppression, for example.) Possible short-term side effects and longer-term risks, insofar as they are known, are presented. You are told which procedures (such as blood tests or X rays) you will be required to undergo in order to monitor the effects of the investigational drug. If you've been receiving treatment with other drugs, you will probably be asked to discontinue those drugs for the duration of the trial so the sponsor can observe the effect of the investigational drug.

What serious health risks are involved.   Some of the more serious possibilities are outlined—perhaps most serious, what could happen to a developing fetus. Strong warnings against pregnancy and/or breast-feeding appear. You are told whether treatment for any injury or damage caused by the trial will be provided or paid for by the institution (it rarely is).

Who is paying for the experimental drug.   Investigational drugs or drugs obtained under a Treatment IND (see Chapter 6, p. 135) are often provided free of charge, although you are responsible for other medical bills (physicians' services, hospital stay, other medications). Under some conditions, sponsors *can* charge for tIND drugs, so be sure to clarify this point.

Exactly what you are signing.   In very plain English and, where appropriate, other languages, it reminds you that you have been made aware of your rights as a participant in the trial, that you understand there could be risks, and that you know whom to call (the physician or a member of the staff) in the event of problems or with any questions about the research project itself. You are asked to attest to the fact that you are volunteering, and you are reminded that you will be given a copy of the consent form. You might be asked to sign another warning about possible birth defects, fertility problems, or harm to nursing infants. Some forms require you to initial virtually every paragraph to show that you have read and understood *exactly* what it means.

ETHICAL ISSUES

Controls

Clinical trials are said to be "controlled" when a group of people, carefully matched to the group taking the experimental drug for gender, age, and diagnosis, *follow the same protocol without taking the new drug.* The control group (often called the control "arm") may take the standard treatment, or they may be given a placebo (see next section). The difference in response between the treatment group and the control group demonstrates the effect of the new drug.

Controls underscore the reliability of a trial. But they are controversial among treatment activists whose concern is that people get new medications as quickly as is reasonably possible. The activists argue that placing patients in control groups represents a diversion of half the possible people who could be testing new drugs (and, at the same time, getting their benefit, if any).

How could the effect of a new drug be assessed without controls? Especially for cancer, *historical controls* are available: Scientists already know the natural history of the disease—what will happen when it is untreated. There are statistics aplenty. The new data (the experimental results) would be compared with what is already known to be the course of the disease. The difference would show the effect of the new drug.

So if all the patients available were on the *experimental* arm of a trial, double the number of people would be taking the new drug. Twice as many people might benefit, and the time it takes to collect data would be cut in half, making needed information available sooner. Of course, not every trial nor each phase of a trial would be an appropriate place for historical controls to be used. But, used intelligently, historical controls could be a real advance.

Placebo

A *placebo* is a dummy pill, an inactive substitute for a treatment drug. Physicians have long recognized that there is a "placebo response": People will often get better after they take a placebo, unaware that what they've taken is not medicine. While this is convincing evidence of the underutilized power of the mind, few people suggest that the mind alone can heal cancer.

Placebos are sometimes used as controls in clinical trials, but *only* in types of cancer for which there is no effective standard treatment. Activists question the use of placebos because there is hardly any cancer that does not respond to some treatment, even if only for a limited period of time. It is never ethically acceptable to not treat a person who has a disease, even a cancer that is not usually responsive to treatment. Even when some treatments don't cure, they may prolong life or improve someone's quality of life. Because no one can tell exactly how anyone responds, the entire question of placebo substitution is troubling.

If you are thinking of participating in a trial with a placebo group, be especially sure you understand *thoroughly* what the choices may mean to you.

Randomization

Patients are assigned to the experimental arm or to the control arm of a clinical trial in as unbiased a way as possible. Randomization, or chance distribution, is usually done by computer. *It guarantees that the treatment groups are alike* so that results and data are reliable and comparable. Randomization is reasonable when the better of two treatments is not known. But ethical problems may arise as information becomes available.

The Tamoxifen® trial presents such an instance. Tamoxifen is a hormone-like compound that mimics the structure of estrogen without having its cancer-promoting effect. It is FDA approved to prevent recurrence of breast cancer, but it may also prevent the disease from developing at all.

As news of this new hope reached the public, there was tremendous interest in the drug. A clinical trial was begun to test whether Tamoxifen could be used to prevent breast cancer from developing in women *at high risk for the disease,* women with a strong family history of breast cancer or with other risk factors. But because Tamoxifen was already approved for one use, it was available to physicians for off-label use also. Many doctors, convinced of its value by authoritative reports in the medical literature, offered it to their own patients at high risk for breast cancer *outside* of the clinical trial. (Remember that it has not yet been *proven* to be preventive.)

Fewer women than expected volunteered for the trial. Women who really wanted to take Tamoxifen got it from their doctors rather than chance being randomized to the no-Tamoxifen (or placebo) control arm of the trial. Unexpectedly, the trial was interrupted in 1994 by news that an unusually high number of women in it were being diagnosed with uterine cancer of a particularly aggressive type. Closer study of the data showed that the risk was increased in women under the age of forty-five, not in older women.

The FDA faced a challenging issue: Does the potential benefit of Tamoxifen—preventing breast cancer—outweigh the slightly increased risk of uterine cancer? Wisely, the agency invited public participation in its deliberations. Advocates, representatives of health organizations, and health care professionals almost universally endorsed continuation of the trial, modifying it so that younger women would be either advised of the new findings or discouraged from participating.

More recently, trials of bone-marrow transplant (ABMT) in breast cancer have suffered similar slow enrollment. ABMT combined with high-dose chemotherapy *has not been proven* to be more effective for breast cancer than chemotherapy alone. But many women believe that it is, and they have sought it as treatment without resorting to trials. As a result, definitive proof that the combined treatments are or are not effective is delayed, and women may be subjecting themselves to unnecessarily harsh treatment. On the other hand, the endorsement that women are giving to the surgery *may* be justified. The dilemma is that, without clinical trials, the benefit of the combination treatment cannot be known for sure.

The purpose of a clinical trial is to discover information. The Tamoxifen trial brought a sharp reminder that using new medications involves risk as well as benefit, but it also demonstrated overwhelmingly that Americans support patients' rights to make informed treatment decisions.

The ABMT situation shows how inflexible scientific ideals can work against the interests of people with cancer. If you are willing to have a bone marrow transplant for breast cancer, you should be able to have it within the context of a clinical trial. That way, you will contribute to knowledge about the procedure. If you have it outside the trial (which most women are doing), that information is lost.

Primary versus Second-Line Therapy

The NCI has concentrated on developing primary or "first-line," therapies—drugs to treat primary cancers. This choice is controversial because there are virtually no drugs *specifically* for second-line treatment, although drugs that fight the development of resistance might be considered as such, when available. (Some drugs are FDA-labeled as second-line therapies but only to fit the out-of-date approval process itself.) In fact, there is little investigation under way into the entire question of how primary cancers differ from secondary, or metastasized, cancers.

It could be important to have an entirely different research direction for second-line treatment drugs because they might have to be different from primary drugs in significant ways:

- *A "recurrence" might actually be a recurrence, or it might be the primary cancer that was inadequately (or incompletely) treated.* If it is a true recurrence, a new population of cells might have to be aggressively treated when preserving your immune system becomes an important consideration. But if the treatment is a "mopping-up" of the original cancer, drugs would have to be designed so that the patient's immune system could be stimulated to participate in the process.

- *Secondary tumors may be very different from primaries.* Over time, tumors diversify into clusters of different cell types. Some cells become resistant to some drugs while others may remain sensitive. In solid tumors, cells on the outside are more readily exposed to circulating cytotoxic drugs, but cells within the tumor are more sheltered. We don't know how to use what we know to get better treatment results.

- *The microclimate of secondary tumors could be different.* The character of an egg changes dramatically if it is in cold or boiling water. In the same way, a cancer that has spread to a distant place is in a different environment. Researchers know that pressure in the tiny spaces around cells differs for cancer cells and normal cells, so it is possible that anyone previously treated may have changes in the biochemical "climate" around a tumor. Minute observations could provide opportunities for developing innovative second-line treatment.

- *Aging or previous treatment can affect your condition.* Overall health and energy are not well understood. Whether a late-developing *secondary* cancer, even five or ten years after cancer treatment, is the same as one that would develop in someone who never had cancer is not known. Whether first-line treatment changes internal chemistry in any way so that a person is in some way different after it is not known. Second-line treatment might take advantage of changes—if they were being studied.

These problems are surfacing because of the successes of a half-century of cancer research. When there were no treatments, no one developed cancers as an effect of treatment—but there weren't millions of survivors, either. Other secondary cancers appear to come from the general failure of immunity in our bodies, which are assaulted by environmental stress and damage. We should actively urge the medical establishment to shift their attention to the pressing concerns about secondary cancers.

Premedication Considerations

Premedication is the treatment you receive to ease the disagreeable or dangerous side effects of chemotherapy drugs. Much better premedications are available now than only a few years ago. But some trials may restrict premedication, which could make the experience more difficult for you.

If you are thinking about enrolling in a trial, be sure that you will be permitted to have antinausea drugs and the steroids or other medications that enhance their effectiveness.

Not all premeds have the same effect in everyone. If you find that what you are taking doesn't work, try another type. They come in oral, injectable, infusible, and suppository forms. Ask other patients whom you know what works for them to get a sense of other possibilities. Determine ahead of time whether it is possible to change the premedication in the trial if you find it does not work for you. It could make a big difference in your quality of life.

Conflict-of-Interest Considerations

• *Researchers are paid for patient participation in clinical trials.* Most people do not realize that it's part of the way their research is funded. You should be aware that this might present a conflict of interest between your doctor's interests and your own.

- *Researchers who have an interest in having you enroll in their trial might unconsciously minimize the risks or soft-pedal them.* You might worry that their financial or professional interest in a successful trial (the hope of ending up with an approvable drug or a publishable paper) will color their interest in your health or well-being. You can minimize that possibility by discussing the trial with *several* of the professionals involved and comparing what they say. Be straightforward with them—let them know that you want all the information, and keep track of it.

- *You might feel pressured to participate if your own doctor is an investigator in a clinical trial.* The relationship between you and your oncologist is complicated by emotions and dependencies that develop around the threat of cancer. In this situation, if you refuse a trial, you might fear that the doctor will become angry or lose interest in you and your case. Nonetheless, you shouldn't feel coerced into doing something you're reluctant to do.

- *You might feel pressured to enroll, hoping that the doctor will take a special interest in you and your case.* Either way, the choice is complicated by powerful emotions, your hopes and fears. If this situation should arise, the best thing to do is to talk about it in a frank, open manner, explaining exactly what you think the issues are.

- *You might want to enroll in a trial that does not involve your doctor.* If you think your oncologist is reluctant to lose you as a patient for financial or other reasons, you cannot and will not be able to trust his or her objective opinion. The only way you can keep hidden agendas from clouding decision making is by talking about them. This situation might present the rare opportunity to reassure the doctor that you rely on your relationship and depend on it for continuing advice and counsel.

- *Your participation in clinical trials incurs costs that you might have to pay.* Controversy about coverage or reimbursement for your treatment as part of a trial is a critical—and central—question. There are more clinical trials of prospective cancer therapies than for any other disease, so cancer patients have a vital interest in the successful resolution of a serious problem. Health insurers and HMOs (health maintenance organizations) are increasingly denying coverage for participation in clinical trials. At the same time, state health authorities are beginning to recognize the need to mandate such coverage, so as not to have a chilling effect on new drug development. It does not appear that there will be a consensus anytime soon.

• *Your goals might conflict with the process of clinical trials.*
Clinical trials define the benefit and risk in a new drug, but the professionals might be more interested in the process than in your goal, which is treatment. Researchers prolong trials when they narrow the patient population to the greatest degree possible. Randomization and the use of placebo or standard-treatment controls halve the number of patients taking a new drug while doubling the time needed to test the drug in the population that could benefit. The accrual of ever-higher mountains of statistics required by regulatory agencies to prove drug safety and/or effectiveness takes time and builds a bureaucracy heavy with statisticians to read and evaluate the data.

These conflicts and complementary interests are pressing issues for society. Because cancer patients are not articulating their needs in any unified way, each patient individually has to do it. People count more than numbers, and the priority for medicine should be treatment, not statistics.

Considering New Directions in Clinical Trials

By far, the majority of clinical trials are tests of compounds that directly attack and kill cancer cells. But increasingly, current studies evaluate new approaches and newer questions of cancer treatment:

How can patients' own natural defenses be strengthened to assist in the fight against cancer?
How can the quality of life of people in treatment for cancer be improved?

All the supplementary medicines that improved treatment, like blood support factors and antinausea drugs, went through the same three-phase clinical trial process as the drugs that kill cancer cells outright.

Some people might consider joining a clinical trial of a collateral treatment because they might be helped or just because it will advance science. For example, there was one small trial of a scalp icepack that, it was hoped, would diminish hair loss while in chemotherapy. (It didn't.) The trial enrolled fully almost immediately because people felt they had nothing to lose—and something possible to gain.

You might consider participating in a clinical trial of a support therapy if it does not *in any way* hinder your optimal treatment for the cancer itself. If it works, you will have the benefit; if it doesn't, you've probably lost nothing—and you have the satisfaction of contributing to knowledge about cancer. Call the Cancer Information Service's 800-number for information about trials of new diagnostics, chemoprotective agents, and other supportive, noncytotoxic therapies.

The Most Important Consideration of All: Your Best Treatment

Everyone who considers enrolling in a clinical trial thinks uncomfortably, *Do I want to be a guinea pig?* The endearing button-eyed creature has endured such indignities of scientific experimentation that its very name stands for squealing humanity in the clutches of ruthless Science.

Is there any truth in the myth? The low percentage of people who join trials is frequently and publicly bemoaned by the scientific establishment, usually followed by the flat statement that research in cancer would advance were every patient in America enrolled in a trial.

But would our interests advance? The real "guinea pig" issues of participation in clinical trials are not about being harmed, which is what everyone thinks of first. They have to do with the goals of research and whether the interests of patients and scientists are always the same.

There is only one important question: *Are YOUR best interests served by participating in a clinical trial?* Because a clinical trial is, practically speaking, just another treatment option, you should evaluate the information and make treatment choices the same way you would if it were not a trial.

6

THE DRUG APPROVAL PROCESS

Getting around the Gate

Most people probably share two convictions about cancer drugs: (1) that *somewhere* the drug exists that will control or cure their cancer; and (2) *if* it exists, their oncologist will be able to get it for them. True? Maybe.

Someplace, perhaps in a university research laboratory or start-up biotechnology facility in your own town, a new agent has been discovered that works against your type of cancer. Or possibly you read about a Japanese or European therapy or even an American drug in clinical trials in a foreign country. You might have learned about these developments by doing your homework—spending time in medical libraries or at the computer, reading cancer journals, combing the literature for word of a promising new therapy for yourself. This one may be it.

Look back at the second opening premise, the one beginning with *if*. At this time in your life, the last thing you want to think about may be federal regulation of *anything*. But one of the least recognized, most crucial effects of federal regulation is its impact upon cancer patients, because the biggest obstacle can be our own by-the-people, for-the-people government.

JACKIE'S CASE

The woman whose picture accompanies the bold newspaper headlines appears at first glance to be smiling, but you wonder whether

her expression isn't more a grimace. She squints into harsh sunlight, a too-fitting symbol of the high-energy beam she is insisting the government should point at her head to kill the cancer growing there.

"A Treatment before Its Time" headlines the story of Jackie's diagnosis, a rare virulent brain cancer, and her effort to be treated with boron neutron capture therapy (BNCT), an experimental radiotherapy (not to be confused with BCNU, a chemotherapy). BNCT was pioneered in the 1950s, a decade of almost unfettered experimentation with radioactive substances. It fell into disrepute after experiments with seventy patients failed to prove it sufficiently useful or safe. By now, however, researchers in Japan have developed and refined BNCT and have reported some success in human clinical trials. Jackie's doctor told her it was her only hope, but no American patient had been treated with BNCT for thirty years.

Any brain cancer threatens and frightens us. Our brains allow us to think and feel, so brain cancer feels like an attack on our very humanity. Jackie is one of 7,000 people found to have glioblastoma multiforme each year, a horrific number; yet it is only one quarter of the total number of primary brain cancers detected annually. The small number of patients and the special difficulties of treating cancers in the brain have made it an unrewarding field of research. Treatments are few, successful treatments rare.

When her doctor suggested "closed-brain surgery" with BNCT, it was only because there was nothing else to offer. But this is no ordinary treatment available at a cancer center. Neutron-beam reactors are controlled by the Department of Energy and found in legendary places like MIT and Brookhaven National Laboratory. Although scientists had made hesitant moves toward instituting clinical trials with BNCT, they were at least a year away from beginning—and researchers had no reason to hurry. But Jackie had a reason.

"If your life is worth it to yourself, you have to fight for it," she said. "It's a campaign for survival." The campaign she mounted had heart-stopping moments, alternately hopeful and despairing. Many different possibilities had to be nurtured simultaneously, including treatment in Japan. Several times, she thought she had everyone's agreement and cooperation, only to learn that the negotiations had broken down. Radiotherapy researchers were reluctant to risk their future work: If Jackie did not benefit (or worsened), they feared a repetition of the events of the past. They were afraid to raise false hope in other patients who were also clamoring for the treatment.

Several government agencies share responsibility for controlling the use of nuclear reactors, and peacetime use has been slow to escape the military grip. The FDA is accountable for research conducted in humans, and any experimental protocol, even involving one single individual, must follow FDA guidelines. (The Institutional Review Board, or IRB, of the hospital in which Jackie had two prior open-brain surgeries had nominal responsibility for the treatment protocol.)

Shrewdly, Jackie recruited the press to play an important role—mobilizing public opinion. Several stories emanating from the Washington bureau of her local newspaper appeared, tracking her progress through the federal bureaucracy. She also contacted anyone who had any influential connections or who knew anyone who could help.

"I'm an ordinary person who pushed," Jackie said. "You know one person who knows another person. . . . I never let go. I learned how to not get no for an answer and to use everybody. I gave them no choice." Her unrelenting persistence over months, telephoning and constantly sending faxes, led her to top federal officials who secured the material and promised access to the facility. Despite scientists' last-minute misgivings about the stability of the reactor, she had her treatment. The very next time the treatment was tried experimentally the reactor failed.

A year later, she had another surgery to clean out the debris of the killed tumor. There was no sign of active disease.

THE FDA: YOUR PARTNER IN TREATMENT

The FDA protects us from harm from unsafe products we might consume. But the same restrictions that protect us can prevent us from having access to new medications when we need them to save our lives.

What is the risk to you of not having a drug available? If a treatment drug is not FDA-approved, it may not be available to treat your cancer. There is a cost to society if thousands of people die for want of a drug that was approved too slowly, was not approved, or was never developed. Overly cautious standards applied to cancer drugs may cost lives because the approval process is *too* deliberate. Laws that are meant to protect may be protecting us to death.

The FDA Affects Us in Many Ways

All drugs that are swallowed, injected, or applied and all devices that diagnose or treat disease are regulated by the FDA. The FDA is an agency of the Department of Public Health, like the NCI a bureau of the Department of Health and Human Services. The FDA is empowered by Congress to ensure that food and drugs marketed to the American public are safe and effective: *safe* means that they will not intentionally harm people; *effective* means that they really do what they say they will. Any product that claims to support or improve health must prove it in lengthy clinical trials.

Except for certain agricultural products that fall under Department of Agriculture regulations, virtually everything that ends up inside a human being, and even inside animals, is studied, tested, and evaluated by the FDA before it is approved for use. The sole exception continues to be tobacco products, although that may be changing to better suit our current "no smoking" environment.

The FDA, frequently characterized as a "gatekeeper" controlling the flow of pharmaceutical products to the American public, is reputed to be the most rigorous agency of its type in the world (there are many). It takes pride in its posture as protector of the American public from the threat of contaminated products, nefarious additives, or useless "quack" medications. Open the box containing a new prescription drug and unfold and read the small, tightly folded, densely printed piece of paper just under the top flap (you may need your eyeglasses). Because it must apply to everyone, it may include extremely rare or frightening adverse reactions and cause you unnecessary worry. Discuss any concerns you have with the prescribing doctor. Because inclusion of the "package insert" is legally required, it also reminds you that the FDA is on the job.

The FDA has authority over the importation of drugs that reach the public not only over the counter but also over the border. Stringent restrictions exist against the importation of many drugs, herbs, and medicaments that are perfectly legal and considered therapeutic in other countries, including pharmaceuticals developed and marketed by American companies that have been approved more quickly abroad.

Why Are Drugs Regulated?

The development of regulation mirrors our concern as a nation for our health and safety. Before the twentieth century, there was no national food or drug law at all. You've probably seen late-nineteenth-century advertisements for the patent medicines, elixirs, nostroms, and wacky gizmos that pervaded the marketplace. They seem amusingly quaint to us now, but they were mostly ineffective or adulterated "snake oils," sold without regard for danger to consumers.

By 1906, public clamor for protection led to the first laws requiring food and drugs to meet official standards of strength and purity. The forerunner of the FDA was formed in 1927 to enforce those laws, but it was not until a disaster in 1937 that the need for regulation became evident to all.

In that year, the chief chemist of a company, wishing to sell the new "wonder drug" sulfanilamide, devised a tasty—but deadly—mixture of the drug, an alcohol solution, and raspberry extract. Two hundred forty gallons of "Elixir Sulphanilamide" were shipped to pharmacies. People who drank the seemingly innocent remedy were poisoned. Not until 107 people had died was the last of the elixir recovered from pharmacy shelves.

Each ingredient alone was known to be safe in the amount used. But because the product had not been tested in animals, the chemist did not know that the combination of alcohol with the sulfa drug caused the formation of a very toxic chemical compound.

The tragedy led to passage in 1938 of the Food, Drug, and Cosmetic Act, the foundation of FDA regulation to this day. It required manufacturers to prove the *safety* of their product and included regulations setting manufacturing standards, tolerance limits for unavoidable adulterants, and other standards. It came at a time of public faith in a centralized, authoritarian government, but there have been significant amendments as new issues have arisen and as the degree of desired government control shifts with time. (As we go through a period of reexamining the extent of regulatory authority, keep that in mind.)

In 1962, public interest was again a critical factor in increasing the authority of the FDA. Thalidomide, a European sedative, was going through routine regulatory investigation here when unsettling news arrived from Europe: Women who had taken the medication early in pregnancy were giving birth to malformed babies. The drug had not been tested in pregnant animals, and the tragic result called attention to the need for special caution in medicating pregnant women. A protection-minded Congress passed legislation requiring manufacturers to prove their products were effective for the intended use as well as safe. Ironically, thalidomide *is* a safe and effective drug against leprosy, still a scourge primarily of underdeveloped countries.

The Orphan Drug Act of 1983 may be the most successful collaboration among the FDA, Congress, and the public interest. It provided manufacturers with tax and patent incentives to develop drugs for rare diseases, those that afflict a relatively small number of Americans. Because almost all cancers are *rare* diseases by this definition, the Act has profound implication for the total, very large cancer-patient population, since treatments for one type of cancer frequently are effective against other types.

Most recently (1994), patient advocates prevailed upon FDA to place its scientific responsibilities above its police function by streamlining some policies so that people with serious illness can have a broader range of therapies from which to choose. "Accelerated approval" brings certain drugs to market more quickly, so the issue of health insurance reimbursement is much less contentious. "Parallel track," presently only applied to AIDS drugs, and other new access mechanisms make drugs available to patients outside of clinical trials. (Drugs to treat AIDS continue to have the highest priority at FDA.) And import regulations are yielding to less dogmatic policies.

If the FDA is going to be made to respond to our needs, each person is going to have to feel personally involved. Because you are.

FDA REGULATION OF CANCER DRUGS

The preceding chapters explained the delicate relationship among drug development, clinical trials, and treatments. This chapter looks at the next step in the process, which has to do with the compatible—and competing—interests of pharmaceutical manufacturers, federal and state regulatory agencies, and patients. It's not a story about how government works; it's about how you may or may not be able to get the treatment you need for your cancer.

How Regulation Determines Which Drugs Are Available

Less than one compound in five that begins the rigorous process of evaluation becomes a medicine. It takes ten to twelve years, 5,000 to 100,000 pages of study results and data, and more than $250 million. Eighty percent of the prospective new therapies are lost to the process as being too toxic or too ineffective. Or they may be safe and effective, but economic considerations may have forced the sponsor to drop efforts to develop the new agent. Perhaps the number of people who could benefit from the new drug is too small to make it financially viable. Perhaps the company did not have the financial backing to support the drug through the prolonged, costly process—a condition endemic to biotechnology companies that are frequently "venture capital," one-drug, start-up companies.

After the Clinical Trials

When the sponsor of a new drug is convinced that the data can prove it effective and safe, it submits a New Drug Application (NDA) to the FDA. NDAs are voluminous documents that contain the clinical trial evidence, complete scientific data, and technical information about the new compound and how it will be manufactured. When the document is received, a "review clock" is supposed to start ticking: The FDA is required to review an NDA within 180 days, a law widely disregarded for its virtual impossibility.

There is no single division in FDA that reviews cancer drugs, which may account in part for the absence of any sense of urgency. Drugs are distributed for review according to what they do. One may be dispatched to the Center for Drug Evaluation and Research (CDER) and then to one of its specialty review divisions. Another may go to the Center for Biologics Evaluation and Research (CBER), from which it will go to *its* own review divisions. Or a drug or device may go to the Center for Devices and Radiological Health (CDRH) for review.

Biologics, for example, such as levamisole and the colony stimu-
lating factors, are reviewed by the Biologic Review Division of CBER.
Many chemotherapy drugs are reviewed by the Oncology and Pul-
monary Drug Products Division of CDER; but anticancer hormones
and hormone-antagonists are reviewed by the Metabolism and Endo-
crine Division of CDER. The newer biotechnology drugs may not be
so easily categorized, adding extra time to the process.

The FDA has many skillful, talented, and idealistic scientists on
its staff. But the fragmentation of the analyses they perform and the
minutiae for which they are responsible have made the agency lose
sight of its unique responsibility: getting new *medicines* to the public
more quickly.

When the review is completed, a public hearing of the application is held with an advisory panel of consultants. The sponsor asks
for approval to sell the drug on the basis that two central questions
are answered satisfactorily:

1. What is the *effectiveness* of this compound?
2. Is it *safe* to use under the conditions of proposed labeling?

The sponsor describes *exactly* how it will be used:

• Alone, as a single agent, or occasionally in combination.
  _____ *is indicated as palliative therapy as a single agent or
  in established combination therapy with other approved chemotherapeutic agents in the following* _____ (lists specific
  regimens).
• In a specific type of cancer at a specific stage.
  _____ *is indicated for the palliative treatment of patients
  with ovarian carcinoma recurrent after prior chemotherapy.*
• At a specific point in treatment (first- or second-line therapy).
  _____ *in combination with other approved drugs is indicated for initial therapy of* _____.
• In a specific rate of administration at a specific concentration.
  _____ *should be administered intravenously at a dose of
  1.2 g/m^2 per day for five consecutive days.*
• By a specific route.
  _____ *is indicated for intravenous or intramuscular administration.*

(Very rarely will an indication be as nonspecific as "may be given by the intramuscular, intravenous, or subcutaneous routes.")

If the advisory panel recommends approval, it defines exactly *what the drug will be approved for*, which is called "the label indication" or just "the label." A colossal amount of additional information also goes on the label, most of which is pharmacological (having to do with the ingredients of the compound and its formulation) or toxicological (warnings of possible side effects). Interestingly—and tellingly—all the adverse reactions, warnings, and contraindications go on the label *before* the dosage information, the risks before the benefit. That is not to say that the information should not be there, nor that what is approved should not be proven. But inherently, the system presents problems for cancer patients, and the problems are growing worse as drug formularies restrict treatment *only to label indications*.

USING DRUGS IN ON-LABEL AND OFF-LABEL INDICATIONS

The FDA Act specifically limits the labeling and promotion of approved drugs to the use(s) proven by the sponsor's clinical trials. Yet many drugs are important in treating several different types of cancer. If doctors were allowed only to use drugs for the *approved* uses, many types of cancer would be without their most effective treatments. But doctors are not limited in the way they may use approved drugs. They can prescribe them in such *nonapproved* ways as:

- Different types or stages of diseases
- Different doses
- Different treatment combinations
- Different patient groups

These nonapproved uses are known as *off-label uses.*
The FDA acknowledges that off-label uses

may be appropriate and rational in certain circumstances, and may, in fact, reflect approaches to drug therapy that have been extensively reported in medical literature. . . .

The term "unapproved use," is, to some extent, misleading. It includes a variety of situations ranging from unstudied to thoroughly investigated drug uses. Valid new uses for drugs already on the market are often first discovered through serendipitous observations and therapeutic innovations, subsequently confirmed by well-planned and executed clinical investigations.

Before such advances can be added to the approved labeling, however, data substantiating the effectiveness of a new use or regimen must be submitted by the manufacturer to FDA for evaluation. This may take time and, without the initiative of the drug manufacturer whose product is involved, may never occur. **For that reason, accepted medical practice often includes drug use that is not reflected in approved drug labeling.***

Why do you have to know about off-label uses? Because cancer is the only specialty for which *primarily off-label uses are treatment.*

Health insurers have deserved their notoriety for setting reimbursement policies against the interests of seriously ill people. They designate off-label indications as "experimental" or "investigational," and they have decided that they do not pay for or reimburse patients for "experimental" treatment. As stated in one standard health insurance policy:

Experimental or obsolete procedures: We will not cover any procedure if it is no longer generally regarded as effective or if it is experimental in the sense that its effectiveness is not generally recognized. A procedure will be covered if an appropriate governmental agency, Federal or (name of) State, recognizes it as sufficiently effective to justify any risks that might be involved. Benefits will also not be available for a hospital stay for such an experimental or obsolete procedure.

Outside of the NCI, which issues information about some *stan-*

FDA Drug Bulletin 12 (April 1982).

dard treatment practices, there is no state or federal body with responsibility to make recommendations, let alone recognize anything as "sufficiently effective to justify any risks that might be involved." The three standard, peer-reviewed, medical compendia that provided the rational support for advanced, nonstandard use of therapies have simply—in many cases—been disregarded. Formularies are lists of drugs that can be prescribed or will be reimbursed by an institution. Your health insurer may restrict your treatment to drugs in its own formulary, or it may not cover you for nonapproved, off-label uses of approved drugs. (See Chapter 7.)

In 1990, the FDA inexplicably used its policing authority to block the exchange of *medical* information about off-label uses. Whatever its motives, the agency provided the underpinning for a general tightening of insurer policies toward off-label use. All cancer treatment is adversely affected, especially for rarer types, because less treatment information exists.

Ben's Case

Ben lives in a small U.S. town, an hour and forty minutes' drive from the Canadian border. He knows the time exactly because he has been making the trip once a month for about two years to bring back medicine that he cannot get here.

Ben has panic disorder, surges of fear and anxiety that sweep over him with startling suddenness, day or night. Panic disorder is a barely recognized affliction, usually relegated to psychologists for talk therapy. Ben considers himself lucky, though, because he has effective treatment: The new antinausea drug Zofran®, so useful in chemotherapy, stops Ben's attack immediately. For him, Zofran is the proverbial magic bullet.

Until very recently, Zofran was only approved for intramuscular injection for cancer-related nausea. When the injection was administered in a hospital or office prior to treatment, patients were protected against the noxious side effects of drugs. But by the time Zofran's effects wore off, the patient was usually at home with only less effective medications to fall back on. There was no oral form of Zofran *approved by the FDA*. It was available, though, in Canada.

Not only did cancer patients benefit, so did Ben. When his panic attacks started, he couldn't take an injection quickly, but he could take a pill. As quickly as it arose, his panic would recede.

Ben's a fighter. He understands that a system is wrong that bars him from access to a therapy that he considers life saving and that the barrier is in place for no sensible reason. He has educated other people to the problems of senseless restriction and has become an advocate of a liberalized policy on access to treatments.

And did his insurance pay for his off-label use of Zofran? Certainly not!

How Drug Regulation Affects Your Treatment

When reimbursement for off-label use of cancer treatment drugs became a problem, an association of cancer treatment hospitals surveyed some medical oncologists about their off-label use of drugs. The results showed that *47 percent of all drug use was in other than labeled indications*. A 1991 Government Accounting Office (GAO) study raised that figure to more than 50 percent, still a conservative estimate. It is now generally agreed that more than 80 percent of chemotherapy involves off-label use of drugs.

A Gallup survey that was sponsored in part by NCI showed that one in eight cancer patients was believed to be *not receiving their doctors' treatment of choice* because of insurers' restriction of off-label uses. Since then, the situation has only become worse. The rise of managed care and HMOs to nearly 50 percent of medical practice has already significantly narrowed treatment choices available to people with cancer.

Several states have attempted to reform the health insurance industry by mandating coverage. Insurance is a state-regulated industry, so fifty separate efforts would need to be made. In many of the states that managed to get off-label coverage mandated, the insurance industry has succeeded in undermining the legislation so that it is not as effective as it must be. Moreover, because insurance is a quagmire of regulations, patients have not become informed about the effect of insurance company policies on their treatment nor actively involved in change. Unlike AIDS patients and advocates, the people most affected have paid little attention to this depressing and destructive situation.

CHANNELS AND LOOPHOLES: EARLY ACCESS TO NEW THERAPIES

As you have seen, the drug approval process is prolonged. But because science is a collaborative process, based on the ideal of free and open exchange of ideas, there is a lot known about any new drug well before it is on the market.

Several perfectly legal (but underutilized) routes exist to help you access drugs that have not yet completed the approval process, that are not approvable, or that have had their approval withdrawn. The various routes have different qualifications and restrictions, and most are overly bureaucratic. Know what you are looking for, and be dogged in getting it.

Some longstanding shortcuts are:

- Group C drugs
- "Special Exceptions"
- Treatment IND (also known as Special Protocol Exemption)
- Emergency IND ("Compassionate Use")
- Orphan drugs

Group C Drugs

The NCI petitions the FDA to designate a Group C drug ("C" for *cancer*) when it:

- Has already demonstrated efficacy in one specific type of cancer.
- Is in clinical trials, but past Phase I.
- Is not normally available to treat patients outside of clinical trials.

Group C drugs are *promising new agents specifically against cancer.* These are drugs still in clinical trials, but there is sufficient evidence that they are safe and effective and "are likely to alter the pattern of treatment of the disease." People who get Group C drugs are *not* participating in clinical trials, and research is *not* the intent.

You must be treated for the *form of disease for which it has received Group C designation.* Any other use would be considered a

"Special Exception," for which there are separate guidelines. (See next section.) The doctor is obligated to follow the standard research protocol for the drug, with the requisite paperwork, although IRB approval is not required.

There is no charge for Group C drugs because they are still investigational. Before each treatment, you must sign an informed consent form, which reminds you not to expect any benefit from the research in which you are participating. Go ahead and play the game.

Only two drugs are designated in Group C at this time, a third, Amsacrine, used for treatment of refractory AML (acute myelogenous leukemia), having been recently withdrawn for lack of demonstrated efficacy.

1. *Azacytidine* for treatment of refractory AML.
2. *Erwinia Asparaginase* for treatment of ALL (acute lymphoblastic leukemia) in patients allergic to *E. Coli* Asparaginase.

In 1993 the NCI tightened Group C regulations so that only those drugs likely to be approved for marketing in the "relatively near future" would receive Group C status. Although NCI credits faster approvals for the fewer number of drugs presently in Group C, the reason for this change and the effect it might have on expedited availability of therapeutics is unknown. There is only one way to obtain a Group C drug: A physician must request it to treat a specific patient. (There is a substantial amount of recordkeeping involved.) The request should be directed, in writing, by telephone, or by fax, to:

National Cancer Institute
Clinical Research Pharmacy Section
Pharmaceutical Management Branch
Executive Plaza North, Room 804
Bethesda, MD 20892
Telephone: 301-496-5725 (Monday–Friday, 9 A.M.–4:30 P.M., EST)
Fax: 301-402-4870

Upon receipt of the application, CTEP applies to the FDA for authorization to distribute the drug for the requested use. The NCI is responsible for and has physical possession of the substance.

Special Exceptions

"Special exceptions" are people who meet one of the following criteria. They are:

- Refractory to standard therapies (the therapies don't work for them).
- Not eligible for participation in established clinical trials.
- Ineligible for trials because they do not have the type of disease being studied.

They are considered special exceptions to the policy of dispensing investigational drugs only under research protocols. The intent is *individual treatment*, much like Emergency, or Compassionate, INDs (investigational new drugs) (see p. 139) without the need to get an IND from the FDA. To obtain a Special Exception drug, a physician must request it. Applicants are evaluated on an individual basis by an NCI physician staff member. An applicant will have a more convincing case if data from the medical literature is provided to show that the drug prolongs survival or improves quality of life. The regulations specifically state that "Reports of low response rates, or responses of brief duration, or anecdotal reports of an occasional response are not sufficient to justify approval."

Requests may be made in writing, by telephone, or by fax to:

National Cancer Institute
Special Exception Coordinator
Investigational Drug Branch
Executive Plaza North
Bethesda, MD 20892
Telephone: 301-496-5725 (Monday–Friday, 9 A.M.–4:30 P.M., EST)
Fax: 301-402-4870

Treatment IND

The Treatment IND (tIND) is a new way for people with serious or immediately life-threatening diseases to be treated with investigational therapies at the earliest possible time. The tIND, also known as a Special Protocol Exemption (SPE), can be used to provide treatment to a single patient or to several patients.

The tIND was developed in 1987 in response to demands of AIDS activists for more humane, flexible drug approval policies. It was the first regulatory procedure to enshrine what have become the basic principles of the "patients' rights" movement:

- That safety is not the sole criterion for people with mortal illness.
- That the possible benefits of a new drug should be weighed against its potential risks.
- That the absence of an effective alternative shifts the balance between risk and benefit toward the benefit, or availability.

Applicants for treatment with a tIND are expected to have *exhausted all other comparable or potentially useful treatments* for their disease or stage of disease. People with both "serious" and "immediately life-threatening" illness may go the tIND route, but they will find that the regulations loosen as the condition worsens:

- In cases of *serious* disease, a drug will generally be made available for tIND treatment during Phase III studies or after the trials have been completed (but before the drug is approved). There are exceptions in appropriate circumstances. Safety concerns weigh more heavily in the FDA's authorization decision if the illness is merely serious, so they are more likely to deny access for serious than for immediately life-threatening conditions. (You might wonder whether earlier treatment might not prevent a disease from progressing to a life-threatening stage.)
- In cases of *immediately life-threatening* disease, the drug will be made available earlier than Phase III, but ordinarily not earlier than Phase II. *Immediately life-threatening* is defined as the stage of disease in which "there is a reasonable likelihood that death will occur within a matter of months *or in which premature death is likely without early treatment* (emphasis added)." In more advanced conditions, the FDA evaluates the drug's potential *before* its risk and then asks whether the risk is "unreasonable."

Treatment with a tIND follows the protocol of a clinical trial, *but is not part of the trial itself.* The trial might not yet be underway, might already be closed, or might otherwise be unavailable to you, perhaps by reason of location; but you would have to be eligible according to the trial criteria. The usual safeguards apply: You are expected to give your informed consent to take a drug whose complete risks and benefits are unknown. IRB approval for your participation must be obtained. Your doctor, who becomes in effect an Investigator under the sponsor's IND (usually the drug company), will have to keep safety data to submit to the FDA and must comply with standard clinical trial safety regulations. The research data is recorded, and your experience is added to the statistical information.

You should also know that although drugs in development and in clinical trials are generally provided without cost to the patient, the related costs of treatment and care are the responsibility of the patient. You *may be charged* for a tIND drug because it is administered outside of a clinical trial.

Because the tIND (or SPE) is a very new mechanism for getting drugs (its very name is still unsettled), if you decide to pursue it, you should be prepared for some uncertainties about the interpretation of the regulations. You will have to be determined and not let yourself be discouraged by bureaucratic nay-saying. There are many unknowns, and FDA policies have developed on a case-by-case basis because there has been little awareness of the new channels of early access. So far, few tINDs have been sought, particularly because physicians may be unwilling to undertake the paperwork required. But undoubtedly, as computerized information spreads earlier word of new drugs, public demand for access to them will follow. We are just at the beginning of that process.

To obtain a tIND drug, your oncologist must first contact the drug's sponsor, who will provide material about the conditions under which it is available. The sponsor might already have a treatment protocol into which your treatment will fit, minimizing the paperwork. If your own physician will be the Clinical Investigator and the sponsor already has the treatment protocol approval, your application will primarily show how you fit the guidelines and explain why you are not in the trial.

If there is no treatment protocol a licensed medical practitioner may submit a complete tIND to the FDA, *after ensuring that the drug will be made available through the sponsor.* It consists of:

1. A cover sheet, FDA form 1571, which provides a summary of the people who will be responsible for your care.

2. Technical information about the drug, supplied by the sponsor.
3. A statement of the steps taken to try to secure the drug.
4. A rationale for the treatment protocol to be followed—why you are a good candidate for the treatment; how you will be treated with it and for how long; how its effects will be evaluated; and what precautions will be taken to minimize the risk to which you will be exposed. (It's a good idea to include information about your prior treatment and to introduce yourself as a *person* to the evaluators.)
5. The physician's qualifications to be a Clinical Investigator, and any clinical experience with the new drug.
6. An agreement to report safety information to FDA.

Treatment INDs are not ordinarily sought by individuals. The application can run to twenty pages or more. There are other, less cumbersome ways to get the same, individual treatment. Instead you can:

- Contact a physician who is part of the treatment protocol.
- Ask your oncologist to become a part of the treatment protocol as a clinical investigator.
- Contact the sponsor about the treatment protocol.

Emergency or Compassionate IND

Compassionate IND—a warm, caring, smiley face of a federal regulation—actually *does not officially exist.* "Compassionate use" is a term employed *only by the NCI* for its own designations—for what it calls Group C or Special Exception drugs—used for treatment outside of clinical trials.

Emergency INDs are authorized by the FDA, which starchily insists, *"These single-patient uses are sometimes referred to as 'compassionate uses,' an unfortunate term implying lack of scientific soundness in these uses."**

Jackie, whose story opened this chapter, prevailed in her fight for access to a nuclear reactor. Although she is less aware of the paperwork that other people did to follow up her successful campaign,

---

* FDA *Clinical Investigator Information Sheets*, 1989.

government agencies are always required to work through already-existing procedures, the same ones available to you and me. Her access was granted through an Emergency IND (eIND), which has its own rules and regulations. She had to be approved (after two tries, but nonetheless) by the IRB of the hospital in which she'd had prior treatment and where she was still a patient.

Emergency INDs provide a way for one doctor to get a new treatment for one patient *facing an immediate medical crisis*.

Drugs are available through eIND requests under certain conditions:

- When a new agent is under active investigation with an IND but is not very far along.
- When a type of cancer does not fit the active research protocols.
- When the drug is *no longer* available through clinical trials, perhaps after their completion but prior to approval (which could be a year or more).
- When a drug is neither under investigation nor marketed in the United States.
- When a drug has been withdrawn by the FDA for safety or other reasons.

In any of these circumstances, *if the FDA considers it necessary*, it will permit the physician making the request to have a new IND for the specified use.

You may request an eIND when:

- You are not responding to standard therapy, or when there *is* no standard therapy.
- You would *not* be eligible for a clinical trial because your case does not fit research protocols.
- You *would* be eligible for a clinical trial that is already closed.
- A new drug is under active investigation but not far enough along to have a treatment protocol for human trials.
- The drug you need is neither under investigation nor marketed in the United States.

The formal request for the eIND must come *from a physician*, although, according to the Office of AIDS and Special Health Issues at FDA, about half the requests for eINDs begin with calls from patients who have read, in the popular press or the medical literature, about some therapy that might benefit them.

You will be asked whether the sponsor of the drug will make it available. In order to expedite the process, you should already know. The sponsor, almost always a pharmaceutical company, is always mentioned in research papers as the supplier of the material under investigation, even if in a footnote. Call them. You may obtain information about individual companies through PhRMA, the trade association for the pharmaceutical industry, at 202-835-3400 or by writing to them at 1100 Fifteenth Street, NW, Washington, DC 20005. Similar information about biotechnology companies can be sought through BIO, 1625 K Street, NW, Washington, DC 20006, or by telephoning 202-857-0244.

Your physician will be asked to provide the following information to the FDA:

1. *Your medical history*, summarizing your previous treatment and results, explaining why the present drug is being requested, for example:
   For two years, Ms. Smith has responded to a regimen of _____ (give details) for non-small-cell lung cancer. At the present time, the tumor is not responding to treatment and has progressed from _____ to _____. Ms. Smith is not eligible for clinical trials with _____ because _____.
   The indications that the tumor will respond to the requested drug are _____.
2. *A treatment plan,* giving a concise—but detailed—explanation of the dose and duration of the proposed treatment, the way in which the drug will be administered, and how you will be monitored for toxicities and treated if they develop.
3. *A statement that you have given or will give your informed consent* to the procedure. It need not be formal or official; a letter from you stating that you understand and consent to treatment is sufficient.
   I hereby consent to treatment with _____ by Dr. _____.
   I understand that this is an investigational use and that I may experience adverse effects.
   Signed,
   _____ (Your Signature)

4. *A summary of the doctor's qualifications as an investigator*, which can be satisfied by including a copy of his or her curriculum vita (professional experience).
5. *A statement indicating the source of the drug* (its sponsor or the NCI), and that they will make it available. You are not expected to pay for the drug, although you will be expected to pay for the cost of administering it and related expenses.

Your physician is obligated to maintain records of the results of your treatment, carefully noting any adverse effects or toxicities. Because you are not a participant in a formal clinical trial, the data that will ultimately end up at the FDA is not expected to be as extensive as if you were in a trial.

The FDA recognizes that, in some cases, moving swiftly can be critically important, so they have made the eIND process work with just a telephone call to 301-443-0104. In many cases, same-day approvals are possible, *particularly if the request is complete on the first go-round*. To save time, the request should be faxed to the FDA at 301-594-6807.

Attn: Office of AIDS and Special Health Issues (HF-12)
5600 Fishers Lane
Rockville, MD 20857

Be sure a telephone number is included in your application, because if the FDA approves it, your doctor will hear very quickly. The agency will assign an official IND number immediately, which will be followed by confirming paperwork. The physician will be required to fill out FDA form 1571 and to include a copy of the correspondence.

The next step is to telephone the suppliers of the drug and advise them of the IND number, whereupon they will ship the therapeutic agent. It seems sensible to request that it be sent by the fastest means possible.

When treatment is completed, the physician should advise FDA of the results and request cancellation of the IND. Should treatment go on for an indefinite period, the FDA may require annual reports on your progress, and so might the sponsor.

Because the eIND is tailored to your individual case, there are specific constraints on your doctor's access to the therapy. It may not be administered to any other patients, and it may not be provided to other doctors for use on other patients. In reality, most physicians will likely have very few patients on INDs because of the amount of paperwork and individual attention required.

Orphan Drugs

Most orphan drugs treat orphan diseases—rare diseases that affect fewer than 200,000 people annually. Some vaccines, diagnostics, or preventive drugs are classified as orphans if they are given to less than a *total* of 200,000 people annually. People with cancer are often surprised to learn that they have an orphan disease. More than 1 million people are diagnosed with cancer each year. So it is not "cancer" that is an orphan, but each *type* of cancer, except breast, lung, and prostate.

Although most cancers are orphan diseases, not all orphan diseases are cancers. Whereas the FDA estimates are that there are 2,000 orphan diseases, the American Medical Association places that number at 5,000. Among the others are diseases like Tourette's syndrome and Hansen's disease (leprosy). Orphan drugs are also used in some addictions, to suppress transplant rejection, and for opportunistic infections associated with AIDS.

There were few treatment options for people with rare diseases until the landmark Orphan Drug Act of 1983. It provided incentives to pharmaceutical companies to foster the development of drugs to prevent, diagnose, or treat orphan diseases when they would have no reasonable expectation of recovering their investment. There is little incentive otherwise to develop new drugs for very small patient populations. In many instances, the disease itself is insufficiently understood for there to be any useful therapy created. And in a small patient population, there might be too few people available for meaningful clinical trials to be conducted.

Orphan drugs *are not FDA-approved*, but sufficient evidence will already exist about their efficacy and safety. An orphan drug may either be a new substance or an unapproved drug used in a new way.

The most difficult thing about getting an orphan drug is *learning about it.* Surprisingly, there is no established way for news of orphan drugs to reach the medical community. Information is spread by word of mouth, perhaps at a medical conference or when a grant program for research is instituted. Lists of orphan drugs are not sent to teaching hospitals or publicized in any way that might hasten the information to clinicians.

The FDA does publish an annual listing, *forty pages long,* of orphan drugs, but the drugs are not grouped by type of disease, which makes it hard to discern when there is something in it for you. The list contains the technical name of the compound, its trade name (if it has one), the indication for which it has orphan status, sponsor information, and more. Complicating the problem are the facts that the list is not often updated and may contain drugs that are no longer orphans.

Anyone can call the Office of Orphan Products Development at the FDA for information about orphan drugs. The number is 1-800-300-7469. (In the Washington, DC, metro area, the local number is 301-443-4903.) The office is receptive to calls from the public and recognizes that patients are often as knowledgeable as professionals. If you call, you will have to request that they sort out the cancer drugs for you under the Freedom of Information Act (FOIA). Such requests are carried out within a reasonable time for a very nominal charge (ten cents per page photocopied). If your physician or a pharmacist knows the name of the specific drug, it will save some time when calling for information. The Office will confirm its orphan status.

Your physician must request the drug and explain why you need it with details that justify the request. Orphan drugs *must be obtained from the sponsor,* usually a drug or biotech company. The FDA can provide details for contacting the appropriate person at the company.

You are eligible for an orphan drug anytime; it is not necessary to exhaust other treatment possibilities first. (There may not be any other possibilities because of the sparse number of drugs available for rarer cancers.) But you *must fit the research inclusion criteria,* and your doctor must *administer the drug under protocol guidelines.*

Because orphan drugs are investigational, whether you pay for them or not will vary. Clarify it with the sponsor.

More information can be obtained by writing to:

Office of Orphan Products Development (HF-35)
Food and Drug Administration
5600 Fishers Lane
Rockville, MD 20857

FOREIGN PHARMACEUTICALS

Import Rules and Regulations

You may want to import a therapy not available in the United States because:

- You read about it in a medical journal or somewhere else, and you think it will be effective for you.
- You wish to continue treatment begun abroad.
- You prefer to take a preparation traditional to your ethnic group.

Cancer is a special case when it comes to so many things. One of them is the whole question of foreign drugs. Rumored cures in this or that distant place arise from time to time; if *only* we could get them here.

In fact, there *are* drugs available, but fewer for cancer than you would think because:

- Drug development is a global enterprise. Many of the drugs first available in other countries were developed by American companies and are eventually approved in the United States. Twenty-one other medically sophisticated countries have the equivalent of our FDA and regulate drugs in much the same way, but faster. Nonetheless, you should understand that drugs that are not FDA approved *might* be effective and safe, but the level of reliability provided by approval is absent.
- Drugs for cancer treatment are different from medication for most other diseases because they are primarily injectable substances. Even their preparation can be dangerously toxic. They must be prepared and administered by professionals here who are willing to take responsibility for them. Most doctors will not risk their

own reputations or your safety on a drug with which they are not familiar.

Learning about Foreign Pharmaceuticals

It is not easy to find drugs that are available elsewhere that might be useful for your own treatment, but it's not as hard as it used to be. There are several encyclopedic guides and compendia of foreign drugs that can supplement what you learn from reading medical periodicals or searching databases. Most guides have the same drawback, though: They list drugs alphabetically by name (usually brand *and* generic), but *not by disease indication.*

So you must know the exact name of the drug for which you are looking. Along with the drug name, guides usually list the disease for which it is used and treatment details; but it is not easy to cross-reference foreign drugs to American drugs in clinical trials or development, which are often referred to by code names or numbers.

To learn whether any foreign drugs are used in treating your form of disease, an electronic database search can be efficient and thorough. (See Chapter 3.) You still have to decide which offers the best treatment possibility, but you will have a comprehensive list of candidates to pursue.

An excellent service is provided by the University of California at San Francisco in its Drug Information Analysis Service if you need information about a specific *foreign* drug's use, dosage, or side effects. You need only know the name. A medical professional (doctor, nurse, pharmacist) must call (415-476-4346) for information from their extensive library of *foreign medical compendia*. Not all countries publish information to the same degree of thoroughness, but they will report whatever is available.

Ordering Foreign Drugs

When you know what medications or supplementary therapies you want, you can order from one of many mail-order drugstores all over the world. It's easier to do in English, so try English-speaking stores first. If you can, you should get a prescription from your doctor. Other countries also have laws regulating toxic drugs, and shipment of certain substances may not be permitted without one.

A list of mail-order drugstores can be found in James H. Johnson's *How to Buy Almost Any Drug Legally Without a Prescription.* * The book has not been updated recently, so before you send an order, you should write, phone, or fax first to check on the information and to clarify payment and shipping details. You may have to fax a copy of the prescription.

Another source is The Healing Alternatives Foundation, which imports many foreign drugs for treating AIDS and other serious illness and for supportive therapy. You might find what you are looking for in their catalog, but you must have a prescription each time you place an order for a prescription drug. There is 24-hour voicemail service for orders, and they accept credit cards. For more information, call 415-626-4053 or 415-626-2316 to hear an informational tape recording. To place an order, call 800-219- 2233, Tuesday through Friday, noon to 6 P.M. (5 P.M. on Saturdays), Pacific time.

Receiving Foreign Drugs

Whether contained in personal baggage or imported by mail, the FDA regulates all importation of medical drugs and devices. Since 1988, when AIDS activists forced the FDA's hand, it has relaxed the persecution of people with serious illness who import, for their own use, foreign medications that are not approved here. For this discussion, *only personal use*, not commercial application, is considered.

• **In personal baggage:** You are allowed to bring through U.S. Customs sufficient quantity of foreign pharmaceuticals for *one person's use for three months*. When possible, it is easier and safer to carry medicine as baggage than to send it by mail.

Only U.S. Customs officers may inspect baggage, but they may alert FDA personnel if they think "an FDA-regulated article represents a health fraud or an unknown risk to health." (In most cases,

*New York, Avon Books, 1990.

this will not be a problem for you. Remember, though, this guideline was *misused* to prevent a woman from bringing a foreign abortion drug into this country for her own use.) If a personal import is brought to FDA attention, the district (local) office will decide on a case-by-case basis whether to detain the article, request a sample for examination, or take other action. They have considerable autonomy, and there is confusion about what the regulations are really meant to do, as well as considerable variation from region to region.

Plan ahead. If you are importing a substance that might present a problem:

> Carry a copy of a doctor's prescription.
> Telephone the FDA about it, and have with you the name of someone at the FDA to mention.
> Be firm and forthright. It's medicine, not contraband.

• **By mail:** Shipments of "personal use" quantities of pharmaceuticals are permitted but are monitored by FDA, not Customs. Unless an "Import Alert" has been placed on what you are importing, regulations require FDA personnel to be "permissive" when:

> The intended use is for a serious condition.
> It is not available domestically.
> You do not take an unreasonable risk in using it.
> You can affirm in writing that it is for your own use.

If a mail shipment is detained, you will be notified with a Notice of Detention and an accompanying letter. You should immediately provide documentation to the office from which the notice originated, by mail or in person, that:

> The product is for use by you to treat a serious condition.
> Your doctor (include name and address) is responsible for your treatment with it.
> The shipment continues treatment begun elsewhere.

Federal Express (FedEx) has a very efficient delivery system, including constant refrigeration for drugs that require it. It's worth the extra expense because their experience with expediting packages through Customs makes it less likely that your package will be detained or get bogged down in red tape.

It's wise to practice defensive shipping by anticipating any FDA objections. If it is not a prescription drug you're importing, you don't need a prescription. If it is, attach a copy of the prescription to the airbill and include a statement with the personal-usage information. If the shipment's value is over $1,250, you must supply triplicate commercial invoices. Any FedEx office can help you with the paperwork, which is a little more detailed than for domestic shipment. Call the FedEx International Desk at 800-247-4747 to make arrangements.

7

MANAGED CARE OR MANAGED PATIENTS?

American health care is full of contradictions. For many of us, it provides on demand the finest services in the world. Yet groups of our fellow citizens have minimal access to care or none at all. Every other medically advanced nation of the world provides its citizens with some type of national health care as a right and benefit of their taxes. Why not America? That question sparked the debate about the need to reform our health care system.

HOW CHANGING HEALTH CARE IS CHANGING CANCER CARE

In an age of rocket-science medicine, we'd still like a Norman Rockwell doctor. But society has reached the apparent limit of its ability to provide unlimited medical services to all, in a personal environment, and without regard to cost. While partisans were scrapping over how to divide the spoils, managed care became the default solution.

Managed care is a catchall designation for a variety of affiliations between health insurance companies and medical providers. Health maintenance organizations (HMOs) are businesses that collect money from you to finance medical care, to organize and provide it, and to evaluate the results. HMOs control costs by controlling services, which means that you, the customer, give up choice (of one kind or another) for the security of having guaranteed access to medical services. There are different types of HMOs, but, for purposes of simplicity, we will assume that *HMO* means any managed care organization.

THE UNDERLYING PROBLEMS: WHY CHANGE? WHY NOW?

Our health care system is, like most of the rest of the world, primarily an employment-based system. For half a century, health insurance has been a workplace-related benefit provided to employees. In our fee-for-service system, we paid into a common fund from which medical bills were paid as they were incurred. We typically went to the doctor of our own choice and made medical decisions in consultation with the doctor, not the insurance company.

Changing Workplace

Now, however, just when economic urgency is pressuring business to reduce costs, the very nature of the workplace itself is changing. Forty million Americans work at home: vast numbers of others are part-time workers at one or more jobs, freelancers, or independent contractors. More than 30 million of our *working* fellow Americans have no health insurance—they have no maternity care, no regular medical checkups, no vaccinations for their children, no mammograms. The inequity is causing terrible strains in society.

Some experts, searching for workable models for change, looked north to Canada's single-payer, government-based health care. Whatever the colliding interests of the various sectors of our health care system, they were united in forestalling the development of a single-payer system here. Yet, recognizing that our own system was in crisis, they had to respond. The present (unsettled) mix of types of managed-care organizations is the result.

Paying More, Getting Less

The costs of health care have been rising at what many believe is an unacceptable rate for our economy. The past few years have seen insurers narrowing their reimbursements and employers curtailing employee benefits in order to reduce expenditures. The following common problems have undermined the security of people *who have health insurance*:

• **Portability** means that you can carry insurance with you from job to job. Many employees today feel trapped in their jobs because their health coverage is *not* portable. If health insurance were universal, they could change employment with no interruption in their health coverage. As it is, there is usually a lag period before someone is covered by a new employer's health plan, exposing the employee (and family) to possible risk. Coverage under COBRA law allows you to continue group health coverage temporarily in the event of job termination, but it is expensive.

• **Preexisting conditions** are medical conditions that you had *before* you were covered by a health insurance policy. When someone with a chronic illness or a preexisting condition changes jobs, the new insurer will insist on a waiting period before providing coverage for treatment of the preexisting condition.

• **Cost caps** are limits set by some insurers on the amount of money they will pay for expensive treatment of chronic illnesses, cancer and AIDS among them. The legal picture is confusing, because limits have been upheld in the courts even when they have been imposed *after* a contract with a higher limit is in force. In addition, many plans have caps on the number of days of hospitalization they will cover.

• **Preauthorization** is prior approval by the insurer for expensive procedures so that they are not overused. Preauthorization may be invoked for routine (but expensive) diagnostic procedures such as MRI (magnetic resonance imaging), but it is often used to deny coverage for treatments that insurers characterize as unproven or not cost-effective. Bone marrow transplantation for treatment of breast cancer is the best-known and most contentious example.

• **Inconsistent regulation of insurance** leads to confusing, contradictory practices. Although regulating the insurance industry is a state responsibility, more than half of all corporations in the country avoid regulation entirely by becoming self-insured. A loophole in the ERISA (Employment Retirement Income Security Act of 1974) regulations that mediate pension and employee benefit plans allows some companies to insulate themselves from virtually all legal challenge to limits they place on coverage.

• **Investigational or experimental treatment** originally referred to new treatment administered within genuinely experimental protocols. However, since the FDA drew some fine distinctions on the uses of already-approved drugs (see *off-label uses,* Chapter 6, p. 129, for a fuller explanation), many insurers expanded their own restrictions to avoid paying for treatment drugs in off-label uses. Cancer treatment has been affected disproportionately by these restrictions because more than half of all cancer treatment incorporates the use of chemotherapy drugs in off-label indications. Several states have responded by mandating reimbursement for cancer treatment with off-label drugs.

WHY WE'RE GOING TO MANAGED CARE

Although HMOs have been in existence for decades, the concept spread more rapidly only as the overall health insurance system was collapsing and the need to respond to a health care crisis became urgent. Some sectors of our health care system have seen the future, and it is managed care. But there are positives and negatives to managed care—it is no panacea for what ails the system. This is not the place for a flat-out review of managed care, but you should have some understanding of the basics so you can understand how long-term treatment for chronic illnesses like cancer is affected.

Given that health coverage is employment-based, it is the promise of cost controls that makes managed care attractive to the marketplace. All managed care organizations have common characteristics designed to control costs: (1) limits on choice of physicians, and (2) limits on access to services.

The "but" for business is whether costs *will* be strictly controlled. There is evidence that the rate of growth of health care spending has slowed for the first time in decades. But with a huge—and hugely profitable—HMO industry still growing, will that money simply be going into a different pocket? In 1994 and 1995, executives of managed care companies were among the most highly paid workers in America, earning many millions of (health care) dollars in salaries and bonuses, their reward for wringing savings out of doctors and other providers and limiting consumers' access to services. It may be hard to see at this point how realistic are the "savings" from managed care we've been promised.

HMO PROS AND CONS

Some advantages of HMOs make them attractive to consumers:

- **No paperwork.** By providing a simple identification card to participants, eliminating confusing and duplicative insurance claims forms, managed care greatly reduces the stressful, time-consuming paperwork required by insurance carriers. The proliferation of hundreds of individual health insurance companies has created a bureaucratic nightmare for medical professionals and patients alike.
- **Access to care.** Managed care plans have many strengths, especially for people who are not sick or whose illness is transient or limited. It feels secure to know that you have access to a physician, for routine or special care, without consideration of cost. The health promotion activities of many HMOs, such as regular screening tests and prevention programs, have offered many participants better choices than they had previously and have resulted in better overall health. Some HMOs even *require* participants to have regular checkups.

But there are negatives as well:

- **Information about coverage is hard to come by.** Glossy brochures about services provided by an HMO gloss over what is not covered. It may be impossible for you to guess in advance the level of services that you will need or that they will provide after a diagnosis of serious illness.

A lawyer who is a survivor of breast cancer and an advocate for patients' rights undertook an informal survey of six major HMOs that revealed that they are often reluctant to disclose information to prospective participants. She learned that:

- All the plans required a primary physician's permission to consult an oncologist, a possibly dangerous delay. When she asked how quickly she might get that permission, only one company provided a definitive answer.

- Virtually all plans require the primary physician's approval of a chemotherapy program. (The primary physician is not a specialist in oncology.)
- All the HMOs had exclusions of coverage for "experimental" treatment, but only three detailed what it meant. All requests for that coverage are evaluated on a case-by-case basis.
- Disclosure of the terms of the agreement is misleading and evasive. Only three companies sent a copy of the contract for examination. Three demanded a binding deposit with the application form prior to receiving a copy of the contract.

At this writing, it is clear that government agencies have seriously failed in their responsibility to regulate health plans and to protect the public's right to information.

- **Concerns about quality of care.** The security of affordable, reliable access to medical care has come at a price: loss of the right to choose our own doctors. How do we really feel about that? What will it mean to us to have impersonal and interchangeable health care providers? Some plans permit out-of-network consultations, although most restrict participants to the plan's network of doctors. If a doctor changes affiliations, you stay, he goes.

Patients and physicians are united in their concerns that cost considerations will drive decision making in health matters. Your access to specialists is controlled by your primary physician; you cannot independently seek another opinion. Days of hospitalization are down; professionals speak of patients leaving hospitals "quicker and sicker." Utilization of expensive technology, such as diagnostic imaging, is discouraged.

Yet, through managed care, many children and elderly people as a group are receiving better care than ever before, whereas people with chronic illness are experiencing worse care. How will limitations on treatment choice affect your health and the health of society? We just don't know yet.

HOW DOES MANAGED CARE WORK?

Managed care is a profit-making business.   Various sectors of the health care industry, the middlemen and providers of services, have gone one further, final step: They are now aggressively managing it, making decisions about how resources are allocated.

Managed care plans are frequently organized around insurance companies. Such large, traditional insurance companies as Aetna, CIGNA, or MetLife have diversified into HMOs, and even the Blue Cross/Blue Shield Associations, which are regulated nonprofits, have formed HMOs in hope of securing greater financial stability. Not all HMOs originated in the insurance industry: Integrated service providers such as Kaiser Permanente, large multispecialty group practices like the Cleveland or Mayo Clinics, or smaller groups of doctors have organized to meet the challenge of a redrawn health system.

Managed care combines features of both insurer and provider of health care. Providing services to a group, not individuals, is the framework of managed care. The group can be small or large; the people in the group can share a workplace, a profession, or place of residence. Cost cutting is the driving force behind the shift. The larger the group membership, the more likely that costs will be contained because the risk of paying out large expenditures is spread out among more people.

Managed care plans might have their own doctors or might contract with independent doctors or even with medical group practices. The plans differ, however, in the degree of control they exert. At the more restrictive end, participants can consult only associated doctors and hospitals for their benefits to be covered. In more liberal organizations or more expensive plans, participants may consult out-of-plan physicians by assuming extra cost (becoming a co-insurer).

Some managed care plans allow patients wider choice. PPOs (Preferred Provider Organizations), IPAs (Independent Practice Associations), and other hybrids are the fastest-growing segment of the managed care market because they allow wider patient choice. Instead of contracting directly for the provision of services to participants, as in HMOs, they have a network of physicians that accept discounted fees from subscribers. At present, more than 25 percent of insured employees are covered by PPOs.

The managed care business is attracting new suppliers to the marketplace. Freestanding associations of specialty providers, such as major cancer centers, are being formed in the expectation of providing specialty services to HMOs. And, in perhaps the most startling realignment of players in the health care game, pharmaceutical manufacturers have entered the managed care market. Several large managed care organizations have been purchased by drug companies in the expectation of enhanced access to oncologists and patients. The waters are getting very muddy indeed.

Finally, a separate group of public payers—Medicare, Medicaid, federal and local employees' programs, and uniformed services programs—complete the broad and confusing offering of managed care.

DOES MANAGED CARE WORK?

In situations that offer consumers a broad range of choices, managed care can work well. Costs are controlled while participants have the opportunity to choose the amount and quality of service they are willing to pay for.

The options available to federal employees, for example, best demonstrate how a national managed care system could work. More than *three hundred* different HMOs compete to enroll 9 million federal employees (there is some regional variability), including members of Congress and White House officials. The Federal Office of Personnel Management ensures that plans are presented and explained in standardized ways, so that the range of costs and benefits may be easily compared by prospective participants. Unfortunately, that is the opposite of the situation facing the rest of us.

Unless you work for the federal government or another entity the size of a state government, university, or large corporation, your opportunity to access good care with flexible choice of plans will be proportionally diminished. The fewer co-workers you have, the fewer choices you are likely to have in your choice of health plans.

In fact, you may have little choice in who manages your care or how it is managed. Your employer may choose the plans and the coverage available to you, and your ability to control the extent of coverage or providers may be limited. Individual coverage is prohibitively expensive; it's better to be part of a group plan.

If you do have choices to make, make them informed choices. There is a mountain of information available about the ins and outs of managed care; there are worksheets, report cards, studies. Do your homework in this, but keep your own special needs in mind.

SPECIAL PROBLEMS OF ONCOLOGY IN MANAGED CARE

In order to control expenses, HMOs and other managed care plans have instituted restrictions on access to care *that can significantly affect cancer patients* individually and as a class. Your plan will probably not spell out these restrictions, but you must understand that they might nonetheless be applied to YOU. As Eugene Schonfeld, founder of the National Kidney Cancer Association, observed, "Managed care is the right-to-life issue of the next century."

Screening Tests

Testing large numbers of people to detect hidden cancers is known as screening. As the public clamors for mass screening for earlier diagnosis, health authorities have actually been *discouraging* use of the tests we already have. Their twin concerns restate the issues that plague discussion about cancer: Are the tests accurate? Are they cost-effective?

The questions are disarmingly simple because the concern is not whether the tests are accurate, but accurate *enough*. How many false positives are there? False negatives? How many people will have to have further (costly) tests to show that the reading was misleading?

Screening can be expensive *for the number of cancers detected*. If every test detected an early, treatable cancer, it would be very cost-effective. If only a few are found, the cost-effectiveness of the test goes down. Economists and others whose work measures the value of our lives against statistics argue against screening.

The Pap test for cervical cancer is frequently cited as an ideal test: inexpensive and accurate. In fact, it gives a percentage of false results, as every test does. The Pap test's economical appeal results from its low-tech origin; it is simply a microscopic examination of tissue.

All managed care includes limits on diagnostic procedures, which can pit the interests of people against institutions. The current controversy over mammography, for example, shows how difficult the issues are. The major voices in cancer agree that women should have a baseline mammogram as early as practicably possible (younger women have dense breast tissue that makes mammography unrevealing). But there is disagreement about the value of mammography as a *screen* to detect very early breast tumors in women between forty and fifty years of age.

Breast cancer activists urge women with no known familial risk to have annual or semiannual mammograms after the age of forty. (In all cases, women known to be at higher risk are encouraged to have semiannual mammograms.) The American Cancer Society supports the recommendation, but the NCI, alone among major cancer organizations, recommends that women with no history of breast cancer have an annual mammogram *only after the age of fifty*. They argue that the test has not proven capable of detecting early tumors in younger women, nor has it contributed to the survival of those women whose tumors were detected and treated.

Do cost-effectiveness questions underlie the NCI's position, and if so, how valid are they? The projected cost of annual screening mammography for the female population is more than $17 billion. When insurers are asked to foot that bill, it is no surprise that they are resistant, saying that it is not effective and that other, manual techniques (including breast self-examination) are useful alternatives. Because it is not yet unquestionably clear that earlier detection in women over age forty *does* contribute to survival, insurers and HMOs have been able to write their own practice guidelines. In many cases, they do not cover the cost of mammograms in women under fifty.

Moreover, controversy is not limited to the cost of *screening* mammography. There are no standard follow-up diagnostic practices after breast cancer, so the annual-versus-semiannual controversy carries over to that arena. Some provider organizations specify annual follow-up mammograms until there is evidence of recurrence—when, of course, it's too late.

Long-term Monitoring

Because cancer is a lifelong disease, monitoring its possible return is a lifelong concern. It is also a lifelong expense. The means of detecting it range from your doctor's cost-effective manual examination to the newest methods that come from the most advanced—and costly—technology. The frequency of monitoring tests and the duration of the testing period (the number of years for which you will be carefully checked) are a source of anxiety to people with cancer. Managed care companies can influence doctors (who might be their employees) to prescribe fewer procedures or to increase the time between them, unfortunately at possible risk to your health.

Childhood Cancers

Most adults would agree that, as bad as cancer is, it's worse when it strikes a child. Yet many children who survive cancer (thanks to remarkable progress in treatment of many childhood cancers) to live into productive adulthood are punished once again. Identified as survivors of the disease, they are virtually uninsurable—and often unemployable. They find their professional opportunities limited and their own families' health jeopardized because of their health-risk factors. The risk? That they will need costly treatment again.

The Americans with Disabilities Act (ADA) is meant to bar just such discrimination, but in many cases it has had the opposite effect. Because more than 80,000 lawsuits have been filed under the ADA, employers have been frightened away from hiring people whom they fear they will not be able to fire. The potential for protection is there, but it's going to take some time to work out kinks in the system.

The Aftermath of Cancer: More Cancer?

New and convincing evidence is pointing at disturbing certainties: that the aftereffects of long-term treatment for cancer with toxic drugs and radiation might be causing secondary cancers to develop years later. The same treatments that are credited with saving so many lives from different types of cancer are responsible for a rise in secondary leukemias, which, moreover, might be more resistant to treatment than the original disease. Because people are surviving cancer longer afterward, they are also developing cancers that take longer to show up.

What, then, does it mean to the employer, insurer, or HMO that faces the prospect of insuring the health of someone who has completed treatment for cancer? Will they be facing rising costs based not on recurrence, but on a completely new medical situation, possibly a very expensive one? Are they jeopardizing the health coverage or cost to others by covering people who are survivors of cancer?

LIMITS ON CHOICE OF PROVIDER

Managed care plans give primary physicians a new, expanded role: as *gatekeeper* controlling access to further medical care. In an effort to reduce the costs of "excess utilization" of services and specialists, HMOs make primary-care doctors the case managers for their patients, with ongoing involvement and responsibility. While utilization (how often we are hospitalized, consult specialists, have tests) has dropped as a result and both annual premiums and annual insurance payouts have been reduced, the effect on the treatment of cancer may be more problematic.

Accessing Specialists

Oncology by its very nature is specialized. Oncological surgeons, medical oncologists (specialists in chemotherapy), and radiation oncologists possess special skills (and frequently board certification) in the practice of their delicate art. Yet there is a trend within managed care to eliminate the involvement of some specialists through the issuance of "practice guidelines": treatment recommendations for physicians to follow, reminiscent of cookbooks. They tell what to do when a patient comes in with certain symptoms or when a disease is under treatment. Their purpose, not entirely bad nor undesirable, is the elimination of ineffective or inappropriate treatment, which would result in an overall improvement in quality of care. (See Outcomes Research on p. 162.)

We consult specialists for their expert knowledge of certain conditions. But if practice guidelines tell primary physicians, who are likely to be family practitioners or internists, what to do under those certain conditions, specialists are unnecessary. They will only be needed to write the guidelines.

The experience of a woman named Ruth was colored by practice guidelines. Ruth waited two months for a consultation with a well-recommended gynecologist in her HMO. When she had called for the appointment, she was told that she would have to "go through" the doctor's associate. Ruth was ushered into the examination room where she expected to see the doctor, but she was examined by the associate, a nurse. Ruth, not an excitable person, rationalized it to herself: The doctor is a busy woman, greatly in demand; she must leave the routine physical exam to the nurse, then discuss the results with patients herself. But it was the nurse who told Ruth that everything was fine and dismissed her. Ruth's confusion was comprehensible. She hadn't understood that "going through" the nurse really meant not going past her.

Ruth asked whether she would have seen the doctor personally if something had indeed been seriously wrong. "No," the nurse replied, "*I* consult with the doctor. Then I advise you of the problem."

Ruth changed gynecologists.

Inside and Outside the Network

Although your plan will have specialists, you may be restricted from consulting them if your "gatekeeper" follows practice guidelines (like Ruth's physician did) and does not recommend it. Some managed care plans allow for consultation with specialists outside the plan's physician network. If you do consult an outside specialist, your plan might or might not agree to provide or pay for a suggested treatment program that is different from their own protocol.

In instances where people have been willing to pay for a different or more experimental treatment, managed care organizations have refused to cover subsequent medical care or even the routine costs of care incurred during the new treatment. By these means, treatment protocols are restricted to only what makes good business sense, which may conflict with good medical judgment or with advanced practices instead of time-honored ones. One cannot accuse doctors of putting economic priorities before medicine, but there are persistent pressures on doctors to make it at least a horse race.

If you feel you are being denied services or access to other opinions that could help, see the end of this chapter for ways to advocate your right to good medical care.

Any Willing Provider

"Any willing provider" controversies are about which doctors join which HMOs. At the present time, nearly three-quarters of all American doctors participate in at least one plan. Should HMOs permit *any* physicians who are willing to provide services for its standard fees to do so? Many do not. They say that by keeping "any willing providers" out of their physician networks, they uphold standards and protect members from inferior or unscrupulous doctors.

On the other hand, many people believe that limiting the doctors who may work with an HMO bars patients from consulting with particularly experienced or specialized practitioners or with ones who are liked and trusted. They believe that this device enables HMOs to enlist the most inexperienced—and hence inexpensive—professionals.

LIMITS ON CHOICE OF TREATMENT

Using Only Standard Treatment

The NCI, through its PDQ (Physicians' Data Query) database, makes treatment recommendations available to all physicians (not just oncologists) who access the service through fax or computer. Similar information is available to patients, abbreviated and in a more user-friendly form. (See Chapter 3.) The recommendations are considered "standard treatment," although oncologists are not bound to follow them. Based on experience, an oncologist might prefer the second-line therapy to the first for an individual patient, might add drugs to a regimen or modify a dose, or might treat for a different length of time.

But consider it from the point of view of an insurer or HMO: If the NCI—the most authoritative cancer institution in the country—is telling us exactly how to treat patients (what to use, how much, and how often), why do we need oncologists? If we have the cookbook, do we need the cook?

The logical endpoint of this thinking in medical practice is rigidity: everyone with the same disease treated exactly alike. Yet it is unfortunately in quite an opposite direction that treatment for cancer should go.

Outcomes Research Narrows Treatment Choice

Outcomes research is the study of what happens to people after they are treated for a disease—how effective the treatment is. If the treatment is effective, it works and the person probably lives a normal life span. If it is completely ineffective, the disease progresses unchecked and the person eventually dies. If it is cost-effective, it works and it is economical. Most results and most treatments lie somewhere in between. Cancer treatment lies *everywhere* in between.

Managed care plans take it as an article of faith that sound treatment practices should be based on outcomes research. They may endorse or deny your treatment depending on the results.

You can see the special difficulty outcomes research poses for cancer, for which there is little hard evidence that *any* treatment is effective or effective for very long. How can a treatment be proven effective: If it cures cancer? If it adds five or ten years to your life? If it works in combination with other drugs but not alone? If it works unpredictably, effective in some people and not in others?

Used alone, almost all cancer drugs are ineffective in prolonging survival. So the answer to the question, *What is the outcome of treatment with this drug*? must be negative. Even when drugs are combined into regimens, or used in an adjuvant mode with surgery, such as in treating breast cancer, the outcome of treatment may be longer survival, not cure.

Should outcome statistics rob us of the chance of treatment, of the hope of survival? I and most people I know with lifethreatening illness would be happy to have more time if that was all we could hope for. The terrible inference of outcomes research is that statisticians, accountants, and business managers can decide that we are just not worth it.

How Much Treatment?

This paragraph appeared in the *New York Times* on January 29, 1995:

> A powerful sign of changing times is a large hole in the ground ... [that] was to be the site for a $50 million cancer center, the kind of showcase that hospitals used to build to attract paying customers. The project was canceled in 1993. The cancer center's demise reflects more than financial woes. For it has dawned on executives here that when you are being paid a flat fee, the last thing you need is to attract more cancer patients.

Most people want every chance to fight for their lives. It is commonplace for cancer patients to try this treatment and that, to go from oncologist to oncologist in hope that the next drug will buy them time—until the *next* drug comes along. Yet that pursuit is extravagant, and more often than not the final outcomes are unchanged. It's just the kind of expense that managed care plans want to cut.

One way they expect to reduce the amount of fruitless treatment is by discouraging patients from seeking it at all. It's called the "no-treatment option," and it consists of explaining the inevitable while reassuring the patient that palliative measures to preclude pain and suffering will be taken.

That half of all people with cancer will eventually die of the disease is a fact. Yet more than 50 percent of us will live longer than five years after diagnosis. The danger for all of us lies in the assumption that statistics *today*, drugs *today*, decisions *today* are static, permanent. In fact, very recent statistics confirm that women with breast cancer *now* have significantly improved chances of long-term survival, thanks to new treatments *administered at least five years ago*. Statistics continue to evolve, and we must protect ourselves against being refused treatment based on out-of-date evidence. We must advocate firmly for the right to have every possible chance to save our lives or to extend them with the benefit of new technology, new drugs, and new techniques.

Selection—Drug Formularies and Off-Label Drug Use

Formularies are lists of prescription drugs that are accepted as useful and effective in treating specific conditions. For many years, three drug formularies, or compendia, in general use were recognized as authoritative: the *US Pharmacopoeia-Dispensing Information* (the "USP" of generic labels), the *American Hospital Formulary Service Drug Information*, and the *American Medical Association Drug Evaluations*.

When the FDA approves a new drug, it specifies, or labels, precisely the purpose for which it can be used and the conditions under which it should be administered: stage of illness, dose, frequency, duration, and so on. But the FDA also recognizes that, when a new drug is released, it is done so on the basis of limited knowledge. With continuing experience in use, more information accumulates about the drug. Often, the substance is found to be useful in effectively treating other diseases or other forms of a disease.

When research demonstrating effective *additional* uses of drugs is published in peer-reviewed medical journals, new treatment information becomes available to the medical community. The three drug compendia cited systematically collect new information, updating their data annually to provide comprehensive resources of "unlabeled" or, more commonly, "off-label" uses. What appears in the three compendia has been widely accepted as standard medical practice.

Off-label uses of cancer treatment drugs are a mainstay of treatment. After all, there are only so many drugs, and so very many forms of cancer. A study by the Government Accounting Office in 1991 showed that at least half of all cancer treatment involves the off-label use of drugs.

How patients are affected.   In an attempt to save money, some insurers and managed care plans have used the FDA's labeling practice to shut off the supply of costly new drugs. Despite the FDA's own official endorsement of off-label use as sound medical practice, most HMOs have termed it "experimental" or "investigational." Because they set their own policy of not covering the cost of experimental or investigational drugs, in many cases people in treatment for cancer are deprived of the most effective drugs for their disease. A few states have written laws to mandate reimbursement for off-label use, but getting the laws written is a laborious process. (Multiply that by fifty. That's why the insurance industry prefers to be a state-regulated industry, although it also takes advantage of exemptions from federal antitrust laws.)

Meanwhile, HMOs, PPOs, hospitals, and others are creating their own drug formularies. The danger is that only the cheapest, oldest drugs will be on them. Treatment may be compromised if physicians are unable to use the full range of effective medication available.

The problem for the public interest.   There is another danger to consider: If the market for new drugs dries up, if new drugs are not bought and used, what incentive will there be for drug development or for research into new treatments? Pharmaceutical research is a function of private enterprise in our country, the means by which the discovery of important substances can generate large profits.

Advances *are* being made in treating cancer. Many people diagnosed today have hope of living longer than ever before, and the quality of life during treatment is better now than it was only five years ago. We used to speak of "drugs in the pipeline" for cancer, but now there are entirely new concepts of treatment, *new pipelines*, that go beyond chemotherapy drugs. We can look forward to genetic treatments, ways to prevent blood supply from reaching new tumors, and vaccination against tumor cells. We jeopardize research and drug development at our peril.

Medical Travel Limitations

Although the federal government recognizes that travel for medical purposes is often necessary and allows it as a deduction from income taxes, managed care plans might not. People with cancer have customarily traveled to consult experts distant from their homes or to access specialized treatment that may be available only in one institution. And, of course, the NCI hospital complex, based in Bethesda, Maryland, provides experimental treatment, if only to those it accepts.

Ironically, participants in many plans might find that they are *forced* to travel. As duplication of medical hardware is pared to cut costs, you might have to travel to get an MRI or to consult a specialist within your plan.

Participation in Clinical Trials—Truly Experimental/Investigational Drugs

The one area that everyone agrees is a problem is clinical trials of genuinely experimental drugs. Insurers and HMOs do not pay for treatment of participants in clinical trials, even though NCI, medical authorities, and patient advocates argue that the exclusion is unjustifiable and inexcusable. Once again, insurers who formerly covered such treatment routinely have eliminated it in the interests of greater profits. At the same time, NCI, ASCO (the oncology professional association), and several private associations of cancer hospitals have adopted policies that encourage patient participation in clinical trials, calling them in many cases the best care available.

While some may disagree, there is no doubt that *clinical trials are treatment opportunities* for many patients who have no other hope for effective treatment. Depriving them of the hope of cure or of a chance of extended survival is not only heartless, it has another, broader effect: It deprives society of knowledge that could benefit the next generation of patients.

Clinical trials are not perfect. Medical institutions have been detached and insular, unaccustomed to considering patient needs. But it is clinical research that has brought us this far. We dare not stop our advances against cancer.

MANAGED CARE ADVOCACY: WHAT TO DO IF YOU HAVE CONCERNS ABOUT YOUR CARE

First, speak with your primary care physician, your oncologist, or the most senior medical person you can get to. If you've been denied a drug or a consultation with a specialist, ask the doctor to reconsider. Explain why you believe it's an important issue and that you intend to pursue it farther. It may be that just a little pressure from you will nudge the matter in your favor.

If you are enrolled in an HMO through a group, take your problem to the person in charge and ask for help in resolving it in your favor. Someone offered the HMO the opportunity to cover your care, and they should know how it's working out.

Second, if the problem is not resolved in a satisfactory way, think of this as an opportunity to practice advocating for yourself. Telephone people in charge, going up the ladder of responsibility until you reach someone who will listen and who seems to be able to do something about your concerns. If you find you've explained your story to two or three people, don't waste any more time. Insist on skipping several rungs—get a senior manager or supervisor.

When you speak with people, ask their *full name* first and *write it down*. It gets their attention and makes them take what they tell you more seriously. Besides, then you know with whom to get back in touch if you're cut off, who told you what, or who left you on hold and never came back.

Third, get a list of the executives of the HMO. You might obtain the information from the HMO itself or from a business library, which will have directories of executives of public and private companies. If you have a problem that is not resolved over the telephone, use it. *Write.* Executives have cadres of assistants to put out fires.

Fourth, if you are denied a service for which you think you are covered, you may need a lawyer. Don't wait too long, and don't be stalled by excuses. It's your health at stake. The field of medical law, formerly concerned with medical malpractice, is burgeoning with actions against HMOs for withholding services. So don't think it has anything to do with you—it's just business.

Tip*: **Demand better coverage***. Why shouldn't you have the same coverage as the federal employees who work for you? Let your Senators and Congressional representatives know that *you* know that they've written themselves a better deal than you can get. Demand the same opportunity for choice and quality care.

8

REACHING OUT FOR HELP

Activism is more than taking charge of your own treatment: It means actively taking charge of your life. Killing cancer cells is only part of restoring yourself to health. *You have to go after what you need in other parts of your life with the same determination.*

Activism draws on the tough, resilient parts of yourself, but it doesn't erase your vulnerability to hurt and fear. Reaching out to others for help and support is an important part of the day-to-day process of living with cancer. Encouragement given and received is therapeutic, information shared can be invaluable, and bringing our fears out of the corners lets us see them more realistically. And—here is the clincher—there is convincing research to show that participation in support groups may benefit patients by adding to longevity.

WHAT KIND OF HELP DO YOU NEED
(OR WANT)?

The kind of help and support you can get from other people will vary with your stage of treatment and recovery—and your own way of doing things. At every stage, though, you'll have new emotional and practical issues with which to deal. Before you do anything, analyze your own needs so you can try to understand those needs with which you want help. Many resources are available, but they will not all help you in the same way. You have to find out what works for you.

If you're just starting treatment, your emotional issues are enormous. You feel disbelief and probably wonder whether the diagnosis is mistaken. You fear what's happening, feeling overwhelmed by the emotional and practical problems that come along with the diagnosis. You cannot trust your body, and every normal twinge or ache is both a reminder and an alarm: What's *that?*

At every stage, your physical well-being is a constant concern. From trying to live normally with the unpredictable side effects of treatment drugs all the way to adjusting to life without a body part, restoring your health will be your vocation, and keeping up your strength and vitality your art.

On a day-to-day basis, you may be tired from the pressure to make treatment decisions, from sleeplessness (from anxiety), and from the extra time it takes to deal with cancer, all of which reminds you that you have it. You're probably spending a lot of time on the telephone, gathering information and trying to choose the best doctor, hospital, or treatment program. It's hard to get away from it.

If you're in treatment, your emotional health should be considered also. You've probably accepted the reality of the situation, but cancer treatment strains the social fabric of life—your family and friends have to learn to live with it, too.

In practical ways, you are likely to be coming to terms with illness, and you're working at accommodating its intrusions into your routine. You structure your life around periodic treatments. You develop coping skills to work out adjustments at home and away from it, at your job and with other important involvements. You could be distracted by some of the problems that come along, for example, insurance questions or significant medical bills. And you may be becoming sophisticated enough to be actively involved in making decisions about your own treatment, which can be a frightening responsibility.

If you're coming to the end of treatment or finished with it, you'll face entirely different emotional challenges. Beneath your joy and relief lie fear of recurrence, fear of the loss of protection that your treatment gave you, and anger at having had to go through a terrible experience. The emotional aftermath of cancer is not unlike what survivors of other random violent threats to life face, posttraumatic stress. It takes time—and effort—to heal from a trauma.

At this point, you are restarting your life or picking up threads dropped along the way. You may have job problems, such as discrimination or "job lock," or insurance difficulties; but you may also be thinking ahead, *outward,* about how you can contribute to ending the menace of cancer to yourself and to those you love—and to everyone else.

HOW JOINING A SUPPORT GROUP CAN HELP

Your Personal Network

Cancer is isolating. It happens to *you,* even though *your* cancer affects the people around you almost as powerfully. And at the same time, it happens to a million and a quarter other people like you every year and to all of *their* families. Support groups have become a helpful way to bring people together to share their experience of a common life crisis. Even if you've never joined a group before, think about it now. It's a tool that can help and that you can put down when you've finished with it.

- Groups help you feel better about yourself by letting you know that you are not alone and not isolated.
- They may help you to live longer by encouraging you to develop emotional and physical coping skills that supplement treatment.
- They are valuable clearinghouses of information.

Since 1979, there has been intriguing, if scattered, research evidence to show that there is a psychological component to longer-term survival in cancer. The authoritative current studies into the value of psychosocial support for people with cancer have been done by David Spiegel, M.D., a professor of psychiatry and behavioral sciences at Stanford University School of Medicine in California. Working with women with metastatic breast cancer, Dr. Spiegel discovered that when they participated in weekly support group sessions, their average survival was *1.5 years longer* than women who did not. And members who participated more often benefited even more in increased longevity.

Whichever treatment they had, people in Dr. Spiegel's study lived longer when they:

- *Joined support groups.* Members benefited in unexpected ways, coped more skillfully with treatment problems, and had a better quality of life, with less anxiety, pain, and depression.
- *Dealt with cancer realistically,* managing treatment, relationships, and their own feelings with a balanced recognition of the seri-

ousness of the situation. Positive attitude has nothing to do with it.

- *Had a realistic understanding of how the disease works* and of their individual reaction to life-threatening illness.
- *Learned to manage everyday stress*, which may free the body to fight disease more fully.

Dr. Spiegel does not say that merely joining a group provides the benefit. In fact, it is not clear *why* women in support groups in the study lived longer. But it is reasonable to conclude that learning to control the mental, physical, and social realms of your life is healthy and empowering.

Most likely, when you are motivated to join a support group, *you are the type of person who is empowered in other areas as well:*

- Taking charge of your treatment.
- Developing effective partnerships with your doctors.
- Supplementing your treatment in other ways that contribute to health and, thus, to longer survival.

You do not feel helpless. You feel your own ability to control your life.

Your Information Network

For people with cancer, there's an invaluable benefit in a group as a clearinghouse for information. Cancer information is notoriously fragmented and hard to come by. The most reliable source may be the person next to you. You'll find that there is a lot of information to share:

Recommendations. Of the many guides to "The Best" doctors or hospitals, none is as immediate as somebody's word-of-mouth rec-ommendation (or its opposite), and you can't ask a book any follow-up questions.

Groups are very good sources of recommendations, and the more limited the group as to type of cancer, the better education you will get in its good specialists, hospitals, and treatments.

Tip: Keep a list of recommended professionals, noting who made the referral. You might need the name later on or might want to pass it along to someone else.

Treatment information.   A lot of valuable discussion in groups focuses on who's getting what treatment, how it feels, and how it works. Pooling information can provide a shortcut to educating yourself about the effective treatments for your type of illness. Become familiar with who has what so you can question them directly and benefit from their treatment experiences. Most people with cancer are eager to help others, and people farther along in treatment have invaluable experience information. Clinical trials should be discussed so you can keep up on the *direction* of treatment progress, the new drugs and the new methods.

Side effects of treatment and how to cope with them is another area in which learning from each other's experience can be irreplaceable. Newer medications are being introduced into routine patient care more rapidly than before, thanks to treatment activists. We benefit from having a creative variety of new types of treatments, but we might be paying a price in less thorough knowledge of their side effects. Treatments can be somewhat unpredictable in different people. Oncologists can only know what they observe in their patients or read in journals, so they might overlook or misdiagnose a subtle or extreme expression of a toxicity—a pain, an allergic reaction, or fatigue.

Your fellow patients' experiences may be a more reliable aid to your own questions than your physician's information. Take advantage of the opportunity.

Tip: If your group doesn't have a library or reference collection, you might want to start one.

Other information.   Cancer-related problems (such as the crisis in insurance, clinical trials, or research funding) that directly or indirectly affect all people in treatment can be shared by a group. If the group is affiliated with a local or national organization or has ties to other groups, you are likely to receive appeals for letters or petitions to be sent to Congress. *It's good for the group to identify itself as a force for change,* because members feel empowered when they are doing something constructive. Keep writing to Congress (or to your state leaders) about issues that concern you.

WHICH TYPE OF GROUP IS RIGHT FOR YOU?

There are two types of support groups: peer groups and groups led by trained professionals, social workers, or psychologists. They are quite different. Think about where you would feel more comfortable. If you have the choice and you're not sure, try them both out until you know what's best for you.

Peer Groups

Self-help groups composed entirely of patients (your peers) do not have a licensed leader or facilitator, although the leader, if there is one, might have had some training in group process. The purpose is (generally) *not therapeutic, but cathartic*, getting rid of the negative feelings that make you feel bad about yourself and your disease—which *is* therapeutic.

Peer groups may be a shade more personal, more deeply intimate, because everyone in them has the disease. The common experience is a glue that bonds the members. Members of peer groups tend to stay with them longer, perhaps because they feel more personally involved or responsible.

Finding a role model is something good that can happen in any kind of group. You might meet someone farther out in time since diagnosis or treatment than you, which gives you hope. Or you might meet someone who has had a setback and has handled it in a way that you admire and would emulate.

There are some drawbacks to peer groups that you should consider when you think about what might work best for yourself:

1. The psychological effect of cancer can be devastating, and members can bring a lot of emotional baggage to the group. A meeting may get too deeply into complex issues or personal problems better left to professionals. If no one present is trained in group dynamics, it could be hurtful to a person whose deep feelings have been tapped *and* to other members of the group as well. Recognizing this, participants in peer groups may unconsciously hold back, being

unwilling to risk going beyond the group's capability, which could blunt the effectiveness of the experience.

2. Groups may have either a shifting population of members who drop in or a more cohesive group of continuing regulars. Drop-in groups tend to stay fixed at a medical crisis-intervention level because most patients come only as they need support or help. In a continuing group, issues are usually explored in depth over a period of time in a more consistent fashion.

Professional Groups

In professionally led groups, the leaders will have a *therapeutic plan* that extends for the (often limited) duration of the group. They have an overview of where the group should be going therapeutically and of the steps it takes to get there.

The most important benefit a professional can bring to a group is the training to deal with painful and frightening emotional issues. In the context of a cancer group, it takes delicacy and skill to manage emotional expression so it is useful—gets to the heart of the problem—but is not overwhelming. Also, the meetings themselves are likely to be more structured. The leader usually gets the meeting started by introducing a topic or question for the group to consider, especially if it is an ongoing group of some duration.

Social workers, nurses, and therapists who constantly work in counseling are likely to have extensive professional contacts. They attend professional seminars and have a wide background. So if you are having practical difficulties related to treatment, transportation, or family therapy, for instance, the professional leader will probably be able to help you with referrals.

While professional groups may be in many respects as sharing, collaborative, and intense as peer groups, there is one important difference: When a nonpatient leader is present, there will inevitably come the moment when the group feels that the leader simply doesn't understand what "we" are feeling. "We" know. Life and death (and everything in between) have meanings different to someone who is facing death's imminent possibility than to someone who knows that natural death will come . . . someday.

And professionals may have their own unconscious fears of cancer or a resistance that can *hinder* the progress of the group or *burden* people with bad feelings. There was one instance when, in the course of a seminar offered to a group of patients, a psychologist offered his view that, for many people, cancer is a turning point that forces them to think about their lives in different ways. Because patients often try to make the most of the time they have ("making lemons into lemonade"), the doctor unfortunately chose to refer to it as "the gift of cancer." Immediately, the audience became uneasy as the breathless leap from "turning point" to "gift" sank in. People murmured to each other, "Some gift!" After a few minutes the speaker realized that he had lost the audience, and he stammered to a conclusion. When he invited questions, he was excoriated for his insensitivity, finally leaving the meeting under a very dark cloud of disapproval.

If you run into such a situation, you should confront it directly, either in the group or with the leader personally. Therapists and social workers who counsel people with life-threatening illness are very special people who might at times become overwhelmed themselves. If you feel uncomfortable about something that happened in a group, talk to the leader about your concerns in a personal way. They will probably be grateful to you for your feedback because they want to help, not hurt.

Tip: Groups in hospitals and social work settings or those sponsored by larger national organizations might have a policy of *staying away from controversies,* such as discussions of alternative therapies or other unorthodox approaches. If you think this will limit your freedom to discuss what you need for yourself, ask in advance about the range of topics the group discusses and how they are approached.

Disease-Specific Groups

A third type of group you might consider joining, even in addition to a conventional support group, is one specific to your type of cancer, if there is one.

Disease-specific groups are one part of the public sector known as voluntary health agencies (VHAs). Most VHAs are foundations because there are tax benefits to both donor and recipient when money is contributed.

VHAs distribute information about the disease and its treatment to the public, provide position papers and press releases on current issues, and educate legislators to their interests. Some VHAs offer services, recommend specialists, provide financial assistance or social services, or have other kinds of direct contact. A few organizations, generally the larger, better-established ones, concentrate on raising funding for research and end up quite remote from the needs or concerns of patients.

If you find a national group for your type of disease, contact it to determine exactly how it can help you (or how you can help it). It is notoriously difficult to get this kind of information, but see the following section for suggestions. Learn what it does. Look at the composition of the Board of Directors and their affiliations. If it's primarily composed of doctors, it probably concentrates on research. Does it have chapters? a telephone hotline? Then it must interact with people. Look to it for the information in which you'd be interested, perhaps educational workshops or support groups.

Request information. When it arrives, gauge whether the VHA appears to be primarily a fund-raising group, an information-and-support organization, or an advocacy one.

If there is a newsletter, try to get a sense of positions it takes— *if* it takes any. The VHA might be an advocacy organization that is expert in the disease. PAACT, a prostate cancer organization, advocated hormonal treatment, contrary to conventional recommendations, years before they were recognized by the medical establishment to be less destructive than standard treatment. CAN ACT, the National Kidney Cancer Association, NABCO, and a few breast cancer organizations publish newsletters that have hard information about new treatments, clinical trials, and insurance developments. Most organizations prefer to avoid controversy and stay on the uplifting side, whereas others simply reprint government handouts. So read carefully and find your own comfort level.

If the VHA adds to your understanding of your disease or contributes to your knowledge or well-being in some other way, *consider becoming a volunteer (if needed) or a regular contributor to the organization.* Too many patients, seared by the traumatic events of diagnosis and treatment, become wrapped up in themselves and feel they should be taken care of. They forget that many organizations struggle for existence and might not make it without member support. Some patients don't think about their responsibility *to themselves and others* to try to end the spectre of cancer.

FINDING A GROUP FOR YOURSELF

When you've familiarized yourself with the types of groups there are, decide for yourself what you want. Sharing feelings? Marching on Washington? Raising money for research?

Your needs may change with time. Your interests may expand with experience. Nothing is graven in stone about this; you're making a choice for the here and now. There are several ways to begin connecting with other people:

Ask a specialist.   Specialists are the doctors most likely to be acquainted with specialized foundations, support groups, and advocacy groups for individual types of cancer. Urologists will know about the National Kidney Cancer Association, but a breast surgeon might not. Many physicians sit on boards of directors of cancer VHAs. Ask more than one doctor—they vary in their awareness of their patients' *nontreatment* supportive care.

Call a hospital.   Departments of social work or oncology often sponsor support groups. Some institutions restrict participation to their own patients, but not all. Be as specific about your own interests as you can. If a hospital does not have social services, ask if they can recommend a hospital that does.

Ask a social worker or oncology nurse.   They are specialists in services provided by their own hospitals and are well informed about organizations outside your locale as well because of their professional associations. Again, if asking one person is not helpful, ask another. Or *another.*

Call the Cancer Information Service (CIS).   The CIS maintains a list of support groups. Call them at 1-800-4-CANCER.

Call a hotline.   Many social work organizations, support groups, and single-disease groups offer a range of services and information over telephone hotlines. An innovation in this type of service is a toll-free telephone Counseling Line from Cancer Care, which provides one-on-one counseling and telephone support groups, as well as more conventional referrals for service. Call them at 1-800-813-HOPE.

Look for **Coping** *Magazine.*   It publishes a list of cancer organizations. You might find a copy in an oncology or social work office, or telephone *Coping* at 615-790-2400. It is the only commercial publication directed at people with cancer. Although it has its share of happy-talk articles, it does offer some solid information.

Contact your religious affiliation.   Many religious groups are working with social welfare organizations to add a spiritual dimension to the physical and mental aspects of cancer healing. They often sponsor workshops for those who wish to add prayer and religious significance to the usual available support. Most hospitals have chaplains of the denominations of their patient population; ask them for referrals, or ask a member of your own clergy.

Try the telephone books.   But don't expect much. Most listings that begin with 'cancer' in the white pages are either doctors' offices or fund-raising organizations. You'll notice that some are listed in large, bold type for the convenience of anyone wanting to make a memorial contribution (which frequently happens).

You stand a better chance of finding a group in the *yellow* pages than in the white because you don't have to know the name of the group you're looking for. In the yellow pages, look under the main heading "Social and Human Services" for listings of Chronic Disease Services, Human Services, Elderly Persons Services, or others that might include chronic disease organizations or support groups.

More helpful is the AT&T directory of toll-free 800-numbers. It has a listing of "Hotlines—Consumer and Public Information," followed by the same listings arranged by state. The list is far from complete, and it's a bit disorganized. Don't expect to call an 800-operator and simply ask for the cancer listings (there aren't any). Nevertheless, you'll find Bosom Buddies in there, and, if you know (or guess) that it's a breast cancer hotline, you'll have succeeded in getting the information you want. Be creative, and look under as many keywords as you can think of. You can find the 800-directory at any library.

Ask around.   As your circle of contacts widens, share information. People are usually happy to recommend what's worked for them. A word-of-mouth recommendation is often better than a professional one, but think about the person making the recommendation. People have different likes, dislikes, needs, and points of view. You may or may not agree with a recommendation (or a caution). You can try something, and then see how it works for you.

MEN AND WOMEN HAVE DIFFERENT NEEDS

Any woman can verify that support groups are full of women—except for men's groups, which are hardly full of anyone. What *is* it with men?

Women and men react differently to communal activity, and that holds true for participation in support groups, even in a crisis. Many studies show that, for every man reaching out to others for help and support in a crisis, *three* women do the same. Most groups open to both sexes end up heavily weighted in attendance toward women. For gender-specific cancers, of course, men go to their own groups, but in smaller numbers than women do for female cancers. And when spouses are invited to workshops to discuss their partners' cancer, fewer men show up than women.

But that does not at all mean that men are less in need of help than women, nor that they wouldn't benefit from it as much. A psychologist, himself a prostate cancer survivor and advocate, in his recent book suggests the dimensions of men's evasion (or denial) when he urges wives of patients to use *any tricks or persuasion necessary* to get their husbands into treatment and into support groups.

Men don't naturally share feelings or look to others for comfort and reinforcement in the same way women do. Girls are socialized early to be sensitive to others' needs and feelings. Boys are not. Women's lives from childhood are involved with other people. Women in a health crisis turn to others for help more naturally than men do. Perhaps men learn that "masculine" behavior is logical, not emotional, and they just aren't comfortable with emotional expression. As a result, men's coping skills may be limited just when they are most needed.

Except for a few specific types, most cancers affect both men and women. There are a few prostate cancer support groups (PAACT and US TOO) and many for breast cancer. The others are nonspecific to type of cancer and gender. Perhaps as men become accustomed to joining prostate and other single-sex groups, the stigma of group participation will diminish. When men reach out for the many benefits of group experience, they may learn to become comfortable discussing deeply felt emotions, even with women present. It could be therapeutic for everyone concerned in a whole new way.

CAN YOUR FAMILY BE YOUR SUPPORT GROUP?

What should you expect from your family in your health crisis? In truth, nothing.

Your family is not a support group. They're too involved, going through the crisis of your health with you. They're just as worried as you are. It's not fair to them, *nor good for you*, to ask more than they can give.

Family Issues

Your family members have their own issues:

- They're afraid of cancer.
- They're afraid they're going to lose you and don't know how to deal with it or talk to you about it.
- They're imagining how their lives will be changed if you're missing.
- They feel guilty about all the preceding feelings.

In other words, there's a lot going on. Someone's got to set the tone for the family crisis, and it will be best *for yourself* if it's you.

Get support from support groups, not your family. Discussing your fears with the people closest to you reinforces their own fears, which can only add to yours. Learn, and draw strength and encouragement, from the understanding of others who share what you're going through. Then bring that courage home without the need to unload excess emotion.

Talk about your treatment goals, not your anxieties.   The aura of
fear that surrounds cancer sets you apart. Nobody knows what to say
to you. Your down-to-earth approach can create an atmosphere for
speaking openly and realistically about the situation, which will be
a relief for everyone. At the same time it relieves you of the burden
of *their* anxiety, it will keep them involved with you.

What you can expect from other people depends on the people
involved. If you have a wide, varied network of *supportive* people,
you'll *all* be able to go on with your lives most normally while you're
in treatment.

Laura's Case

Laura is from South Carolina, the youngest daughter of a traditional
southern family. Her father had prostate cancer three years before
Laura's colon cancer was discovered, ten years ago. His treatment
consisted of twenty-eight courses of radiation, during which time
Laura's mother kept her anxieties in check by constant reassurance
from his doctor. At the end of the treatment, bone scans showed he
was all right.

Life in the South is rooted in its own history: There is a sense
of—and a search for—the continuity in life's events and an orderly
way of approaching them. Laura's treatment was appropriate to her
own case, but her mother would burden her with persistent questions
and instructions. As she neared the end of treatment, her mother constantly asked her when she was going to have her bone scans. "They
did it for Dad. Why not you?" she asked.

Laura recognized that she couldn't help her mother have insight
into the nature of cancer treatment. She learned instead to deflect
unanswerable questions by saying, "Mother, now I'm going to call
you back in three days, and we'll talk again." And she would hang
up. Her own survival was at stake. "One of the hardest things is to
sort out what you have to do to save yourself. The energies of my life
had to go to me," she says.

One of her older sisters has never discussed her illness with her,
to Laura's great disappointment. "In my heart I knew that bitterness
wouldn't help me. I had to get beyond it, to forgiveness and understanding."

The need to protect family members can be a burden, but it's one
we really have no choice about accepting.

POST-TREATMENT SURVIVORS' GROUPS: A DIFFERENT AGENDA

The concerns, issues, and frustrations of people in treatment are similar and related, but what faces people who have *finished* treatment is separate—and very different.

Only now, when there is a large number of long-term survivors of both childhood and adult cancers are their special needs becoming recognized. The burgeoning of post-treatment support groups is an encouraging development, which will surely contribute to the survivors' well-being.

Survivors' Issues

Survivors' groups have a distinct agenda:

Restarting your life.   Everyone in ongoing treatment for cancer organizes their lives around it. It's as if the every-three-week chemotherapy or every-day radiation restarts your clock; everything else follows it. But immediately following completion of active treatment, life has to be restructured. It can feel oddly as if something is missing.

It's very helpful to share problems with other people going through the same transitional experiences, such as getting family and other relationships back on a more normal (less guarded) footing, and "learning to smell the roses," taking pleasure in all the things in your life without the special intensity given it by being in treatment.

Facing the aftermaths.   Given the bewildering variety of cancers and the dramatic interventions of which medicine is capable, thousands of people are surviving cancer only to be left handicapped to some degree. Disability can take the form of psychological scars (and who *doesn't* have those after cancer), physical scars that are not normally visible, and other physical effects, such as the loss of a body part or infertility. Physical and emotional aftermaths of the disease have consequences that can affect family relationships, work situations, and other terribly important aspects of our lives.

Survivors can help each other in the sensitive period of coming to terms with *having a future again*. Self-image, self-esteem, and self-confidence are often damaged by the depersonalization of treatment. They can be repaired. The experience of the disease makes almost everyone more perceptive of others with cancer, so while joining a group will help you, you will be helping other people.

Managing the practical consequences.   Some of the most serious follow-up problems faced by people after cancer are also among the least likely to change. You may feel locked into your job because of insurance restrictions. Your insurance company may be less than cooperative or even threatening. You might feel you are being discriminated against in your job because of your health.

Although there are no easy answers to these perplexing difficulties, you may learn how other people handled similar situations, or you may help others toward their own solutions from your experience. Too many people expect to pick up the telephone and find someone *else* available to provide a solution. I well remember a woman who called CAN ACT to help her with an insurance problem. When I explained that we are a public policy organization that advocates the empowerment of patients *to help themselves*, she was very indignant. "You should call yourselves 'CAN'T ACT,' " she snorted, and hung up.

Living with fear of recurrence.   Cancer is a life-changing illness and surviving is a lifelong process. Graduating to a survivors' group doesn't come with guarantees.

Relapse and recurrence are facts of cancer we always knew were possible. But a newly recognized phenomenon is the development of recurrences or secondary tumors in long-term survivors as a delayed effect of treatment for the earlier cancer. This has caused alarm in the medical community, to say nothing of its effect on the patient community: It means that we are at risk forever.

A nurse who herself had breast cancer twenty years after Hodgkin's disease recommends that oncologists have an "exit interview" with patients on completion of treatment to advise that the risk of secondary cancer may *increase* with time from the primary. It certainly means that prudent patients will maintain a lifelong association with their oncologists.

So, finally, we have to learn to live with the ironic fact that successful treatment brings with it the probability of more cancer.

Learning to trust your body.   Your body betrayed you by becoming ill. It's natural to feel vulnerable, to fear that you can never rely on your health again. It takes time because you've been through regimens that strained every resource you had; but it *is* possible.

You'll find yourself feeling better and stronger, developing a sense of health and well-being *with time.* You may only be able to gauge how much better you feel by *looking back* to how you felt while you were in treatment: fatigued, achy, sick, possibly with a host of side effects. If a post-treatment group has members who are farther out from treatment, listen to how issues change and priorities normalize. It will happen to you, too.

A Model Post-Treatment Program

The Post-Treatment Resource Program (PTRP) at Memorial Sloan-Kettering Cancer Center in New York City is an innovative resource for patients who have finished active treatment. This metropolitan cancer hospital has a mental health component integrated into its active treatment programs. The skilled counseling staff saw a natural opportunity to extend it to an after-care service for an underserved population.

PTRP is multidisciplinary, providing education, guidance, and peer support to the hospital's own patients as well as to the public at large. The hospital's medical staff and others are invited to give seminars, which brings doctors and patients together in a more informal setting; it holds workshops on diverse topics and maintains a resource library. There are both peer-led and guided support groups, and individual counseling is available. Open-house meetings on subjects of general interest attract people from all parts of the city, while a year-end holiday party bonds participants, their families, and PTRP's staff in an annual shared celebration of life.

Some of the activities are free, although participants are asked to contribute a nominal fee for other activities. Costs for individual and group counseling follow established hospital policy, but they are modified in cases of financial hardship.

PTRP has an active outreach program, which sets Sloan-Kettering apart from other institutions with a more hands-off attitude. Program announcements are posted in public spaces in the hospital, and medical staff are asked for patient referrals. In addition, a computer database of patients who have recently completed treatment is consulted, and, after evaluation with physicians for appropriateness, the "graduates" of treatment are invited to participate.

Since the program began in 1988, it has grown dramatically, testament to people's need for knowledge, help, and a supportive environment in the long post-treatment period.

Is a resource like PTRP available to you? If you are at the time in treatment when you are looking for the kind of help it provides, begin with the largest cancer treatment hospital within your area. It is likely to have the greatest number of patients, the most diverse social work department, and the resources to provide quality-of-life services. If they only have support groups for ongoing patients, suggest they start a post-treatment program.

Other hospitals or specialized social work resources (such as Cancer Care in New York, New Jersey, and Connecticut) might already have or might be interested in forming post-treatment groups. If you do not succeed in finding one, contact the American Cancer Society (800-ACS-2345) or the National Coalition for Cancer Survivorship (301-650-8868) to see whether they provide services in your area. The latter group has a newsletter that matches patients for self-help when a group cannot be found or formed. Y-ME, a national breast cancer organization, has many chapters with support groups. If they do not have a chapter in your area, they will refer you appropriately (800-221-2141).

STARTING YOUR OWN SUPPORT GROUP

You may find, after doing the research, that no convenient support group meets your needs. Perhaps you are looking for people with the same type of disease or have a different agenda from the services available. Maybe you simply have a time conflict.

The idea of starting your own group may cross your mind, but you don't know whether an undertaking like that is doable or unrealistic. In fact, grassroots self-help organizations are an American tradition. If you can *define your goals and limits*, you can form a support group that will best fit your own needs.

What Do You Want from a Group?

You might want to meet others with your specific disease or people at the same stage of treatment. You might be interested in building a network of caring friends for mutual support and encouragement. Or you might be more interested in exchanging survival strategies so you can get more information about treatments and medical developments related to your common disease. Decide whether you think a professional (therapist or social worker) should lead the group because the practical results are quite different.

Be sure you understand your own goals. If you're going to the trouble of organizing a group (and it involves some of your time, energy, and money), it's got to meet your needs first.

How Much Are You Willing to Do?

Set limits for yourself. You're probably not interested in reinventing the American Cancer Society at this point in your life. If you want a small, intimate group that meets in members' homes, you'll go about starting it differently than if you were setting up a crisis hotline or a nonprofit organization. The commitment and the amount of work involved in starting *anything*, no matter how small, is always greater than you imagine. Don't get in over your head.

Who Will Join the Group?

To assess whether there is interest in your idea of a group, prepare a flyer that you will distribute no more than two to three weeks in advance of a meeting date. State that it is a first meeting, and define clearly the group to which you are speaking. Write down some of the topics you think are important for discussion, in such a way that will catch the interest of other people with the same concerns.

You're likely to get a better response if you include your telephone number and a mailing coupon or little tear-offs across the bottom of the page with your phone number. When people cannot attend the first meeting, they can indicate that they are interested in participating in a future meeting. *Capture the name and address of everyone who shows interest.* It can be the basis of a future mailing list.

Distribute the flyer anywhere a potential member might run across it. Hospitals' oncology and social work departments are particularly appropriate because that's where the patients are. Naturally you'll discuss what you're doing with the professional staff, which may be willing to refer people to you. Clergymen, oncologists, hematologists, and others in private practices who work with people with cancer are good sources. Post the flyer in public spaces, such as on community bulletin boards in malls, supermarkets, libraries, and schools.

Ask community-based newspapers if they will run the flyer as a small-space ad on a pro bono basis (as a public service, for free), or place an announcement in a "community events" column of a local newspaper.

When you start to get a response, as you should, explain what you are doing and why. Ask everyone to spread the word to their friends. Don't be discouraged if only a few show up. Men *and* women with cancer are notorious for not participating. It's part of the problem of our feeling little control over our own survival. It's not personal, and it's not about you. It's about cancer.

Planning the First Meeting

Prepare an agenda for the meeting. Don't get in over your head with too tight a plan. A good way to establish a bond: Ask for *brief* personal histories and then ask everyone what they expect from the group. The group should decide what limits it wants to set on discussion topics: Should it include discussion of alternative (herbal, homeopathic, or nontoxic) anticancer agents and meditation? Should it listen to self-awareness tapes? Should discussion be restricted to personal experiences? Or should it combine all self-help modalities? People who might join the group in the future are affected by the decisions you make now.

Think about a second meeting in advance. If enough interested people come to the first meeting, you'll surely have a second one. If you don't want to find yourself permanently doing all—or most—of the work, plan that the second meeting will be organizational. Dividing up the work and responsibility will involve people in the group's activities in a meaningful way. Try to gauge who might volunteer for leadership roles or who might be assigned responsible positions.

Plan to enlarge the scope of the group.   A wonderful way to build public awareness of and support for a new group is to have a public event to let people know you're there. Doctors are always a big draw as speakers, especially if they are willing to talk about treatments or nutrition and to *answer questions afterward.* The opportunity to get off-the-cuff medical opinions is an irresistible draw and usually attracts larger numbers of interested people.

Or, if it fits the group style, think about having a rally. Although a rally connotes activism, under certain conditions it can be about sharing and gathering support, rather than politics. Mother's Day has become a day for focusing on breast cancer activities in many parts of the country. *Coping* magazine sponsors a National Cancer Survivors' Day (contact them for details) in which many local hospitals participate. You might have a table with information, your flyers, and (always) a sign-up sheet. How about Father's Day for men's cancer activities? Establishing a support group is as much an empowering activity as any other.

Preparing for a public meeting takes a lot of preparation but not enough to scare you off. Make sure you keep everyone involved by thinking of different ways to use their participation. *Don't let anyone go away without an assignment*—it's a way to keep them involved. One person can find the speaker, another can solicit funds for a coffee hour before or after the meeting, a third can find a public space to be donated for the meeting, and so on.

Tip: Try to involve local politicians. They like to be associated with things that make them look good, and they have contacts that you can use.

Make some longer-range plans.   Should the group become affiliated with a hospital? It would put you in touch with groups of people who might become new members, but disadvantages include the need to defer to institutional policies. If the group's agenda includes discussion of heavy emotional matters, you would be wise to consider how to gain the participation of a social worker or therapist or even of a trained peer counselor. As the scale of your thinking expands, you might consider involving a skilled organizer, a fund-raiser, and a publicity person. These are difficult—but not impossible—tasks for volunteers.

9

THE EMPOWERED PATIENT
Doing Something about Cancer

"Activists are ordinary people doing extraordinary things," stated one anonymous source. This book has tried to convince you that you will *feel* better and *do* better when you participate in making decisions about your treatment, when you become the expert in your own case. Because we all live in a society that has feelings about cancer and about people with cancer, we have to learn for ourselves where we fit into the larger picture so we can be effective in changing things for ourselves and others.

THREE AGENDAS FOR CANCER

The Personal Agenda

We fight cancer on many levels.

The first level is the most intimate and urgent, confined to the space of our bodies. It's our personal fight against physical disease.

The Social Agenda

The second level, like a medium-size box that encloses the smaller box of the personal fight, is the *environment* in which we're fighting cancer. It involves the people around us who offer support, information, and help in our ongoing battle.

Your empowerment, like your disease, doesn't take place in a vacuum, but in a society that shapes the conditions that can support your personal growth while you're trying to get back your health.

The Political Agenda

The largest box, containing the other two, is the larger context of cancer, how *your* cancer is part of what "cancer" means to society. And it's the one in which you don't *get* anything—you *give*.

Give what? During treatment, few people think about their cancer in any larger context because active disease is a crisis. But they don't think about it that way when their treatment is finished either. They don't know that they can give something back that might benefit them again years later.

BEYOND SURVIVING

The time will come when you are out of treatment or when treatment has become integrated into your life so you can gain perspective on what you've been through.

There's nothing like life-threatening illness to teach us one supreme lesson: that we *really* have little control over our lives and little power over what befalls us. Great and powerful people die of cancer every day, unable to buy or command health any more than you or I can.

Activating Cancer Survivors

In spite of the impact of cancer on the American public in every way measureable (one in three families affected, years of productivity lost to the economy, and so on), there has not been a sense of urgency to find the origin of cancer, to find new ways of treating it, and to devise strategies to prevent it from developing. Do you really *believe* the answer is broccoli? Look, by contrast, at the public attitude toward AIDS, which overall affects one-tenth the number of people who get cancer each year: We have come to act as if AIDS is a "cause" (a movement) and cancer is only a disease.

Why is that?

• Cancer is a *professional* concern. The people making policy decisions about cancer are doctors, researchers, and even technicians; oncology nurses and social workers; executives of drug companies and of health insurance companies; fund-raisers and lobbyists. These are the people sitting on hospital boards and pharmaceutical company boards, the board of the American Cancer Society, the boards of the hundreds of smaller fund-raising organizations. Is it any wonder there's no sense of urgency about your life or mine?

• Those of us with cancer have no sense of ourselves as members of a group. Cancer is isolating, not communal. There are many differences between the AIDS and cancer populations, but we could learn a few lessons in empowerment from them.

Surviving cancer yourself is not enough. It's not doing enough. You know now that the threat or the reality of it will be with you for the rest of your life. If you want to change that for yourself, or lessen the threat for those you love, *you* must get involved in changing what we do and how we think about cancer.

Gene

While Gene was hospitalized for the removal of a cancerous kidney, he received an invitation to the first meeting of a kidney cancer support group put together by an oncologist he had once consulted. He saved the information, and, by the group's third meeting, Gene was sufficiently recovered to join.

"People sat around telling medical war stories," he recounts, "wringing their hands and bemoaning the facts of kidney cancer." Gene is a businessman who holds an advanced degree in business management. He has a confident, matter-of-fact manner. "I said, 'I'm leaving. When you want to *do something* about it, call me.'"

That got the others' attention because they believed that there really was nothing to be done, that they came together in groups to cry, to share feelings, and to give each other "support"—and go home.

"Do what?" they asked. Gene said, "This is a free country. We can start a specialized hospital, start a national organization, do whatever we want."

That night, the National Kidney Cancer Association was born. Gene and several others developed an ambitious strategic plan—to improve care, increase survival, inform and educate patients and the public, sponsor research, and act as an advocate on behalf of patients.

The new organization, with Gene as president, quickly published the first useful patient brochure about the disease. It was called *We Have Kidney Cancer* and was funded by drug companies that have an interest in the treatment of kidney cancer. It was widely distributed to urologists and oncologists. The number of people who get kidney cancer is relatively small, which makes the question of which cancer research is funded, encouraged, and approved sharply pointed.

Since its founding more than five years ago, the NKCA has become a significant force in cancer policy, largely because Gene himself is a significant force. The organization has granted research funds, fostered productive clinical trials, and effectively pressed both Congress and the FDA for progressive change. It has chapters in several cities, has had three annual conventions, and is among the best informed, most effective patient organizations in existence.

And it all started with one person.

CANCER AND AIDS ACTIVISM

What AIDS Activism Can Teach Us

The most basic difference between people with cancer and people with HIV and/or AIDS (here abbreviated only as AIDS) is that those with AIDS recognize that they are part of a relatively small, disproportionately powerful special-interest group.

Those of us with cancer, on the other hand, do *not* identify ourselves as part of a special-interest group. As a result, we are members of a group with power disproportionately *small* to our vast numbers.

A decade into the AIDS epidemic, the number of drugs approved to treat HIV- and AIDS-related conditions in recent years is about equal to that for cancer, a breathtaking statistic. On the basis of number of people affected alone, there should be at least *ten times* the number of drugs for cancer as AIDS. The numbers show you that pressure from a motivated interest group *can* drive research to be more focused and more productive. They show you that government funding *can* be directed and that regulatory agencies *can* be made to respond to the needs of people, not paperwork. The success of AIDS activists should show you what we could do if we thought about ourselves as a powerful special-interest group.

How Cancer Is Different from AIDS Activism

Cancer activism is a whisper next to the amplified voice of AIDS for reasons that begin in every patient on the day of diagnosis. How we see ourselves as people with a disease affects what we ultimately think we can do about it.

People with cancer are isolated by their illness.   When people are diagnosed with cancer, it is usually a medically acute situation. They are plunged into invasive treatment that frequently makes them feel worse than they did before the diagnosis. Especially at the beginning of treatment, they cannot reasonably be expected to take an activist role in public policy matters.

At the present time, HIV may be diagnosed years before the onset of AIDS. Most AIDS activists are HIV-positive but still healthy enough to be involved in social activism. They are motivated, even driven, by awareness of their own health issues as well as those of others close to them.

The social structures of cancer reinforce dependency.   The services available to people with cancer are primarily psychosocial and supportive. They help patients adjust to the disease and treatment, but very few encourage more direct intervention. Some grassroots breast cancer organizations do take a variety of approaches to public policy issues that offers choices to the would-be activist. But if someone were motivated to work on behalf of esophageal cancer, the choices available would be zero to nonexistent.

AIDS organizations run the gamut from militantly confrontational groups to mainstream, conservative equivalents of the ACS. Anyone who looks for it can probably find a good fit in AIDS activism.

People with cancer have psychological barricades.   Cancer patients depend on their doctors, not on each other or themselves. Dependency disempowers us. Relatively few people question doctors; fewer still question the cancer establishment. So if someone runs into a problem getting a treatment, it is rare to think that the system is wrong and that the person *can and should* do something about it. It is more rare still that the friends and family of the patient believe they have the *ability and responsibility* to do something also.

On the other hand, we all know how effective AIDS activism has been in convincing society that the disease is *everyone's* responsibility. Entire industries (entertainment and fashion, for two) compete to become identified with AIDS. Sports figures vying for elevation to heroic status announce their HIV status almost smugly. Which celebrities have you heard about lately that are doing anything for cancer (except maybe planning to "beat it" themselves)?

Why Is Cancer Activism Weak?

Cancer activism is weak and disempowered because patients do not believe they can be strong. The development of breast cancer advocacy shows, however, how determined activists can change that. Long-overdue attention—and significant levels of research funding and talent—is finally being directed at breast cancer, thanks to skillful political maneuvers by newly unified breast cancer organizations. (The benefit does not flow to other cancers.)

Founding the National Breast Cancer Coalition

Unique conditions led to the founding of a national advocacy organization for breast cancer, but other cancer organizations can learn from those conditions and apply them to advocacy for other types of cancer.

- There were enormous numbers of patients: In 1993, one woman in nine (now eight) could expect to have the disease in her lifetime, up from *one in twenty* a few decades before. Breast cancer is one of the most frequently diagnosed cancers, second only to lung.
- Facts were becoming known about the even more shocking incidence of breast cancer in lesbian women (one in three), galvanizing a movement among them for some way to brake the accelerating incidence of the disease.
- Support groups for women with breast cancer already peppered the landscape, from professional ones sponsored by institutions as vast as the ACS to informal self-help groups meeting in

women's homes in small towns all over America. As the coalition developed, these groups were gradually drawn into it by a series of petition campaigns that sought to capture every interested individual.

• There was pressure for more attention to women's health in general, which had been neglected at the highest levels of government-sponsored research. There was astonishing lack of knowledge about the basic biology of breast cancer, about cardiovascular disease in women, and about other life-threatening illnesses. Advocates frequently cited the fact that they were being treated with the same regimens as women had been a generation prior because of the stagnation in research.

The first meetings of what was to become the nucleus of the National Breast Cancer Coalition (NBCC) included only a few organizations, among which was CAN ACT. Subsequent meetings with an ever-expanding spectrum of breast cancer organizations led to the founding of the national organization. One of the early decisions was to make the NBCC a lobby, as opposed to a nonprofit, identifying Congress as the source of policies that affected breast cancer (through its power to allocate resources) and so directly seeking to influence it. Another was to immediately retain an "insider" Washington public-relations firm identified with women's issues, which smoothly integrated the new organization into the Washington circuit.

The NBCC has been very successful. It has made breast cancer respected and sufficiently feared that members of Congress hesitate before cutting research budgets to consider the consequences to their own employment prospects (just as they do for AIDS). Most important, the NBCC has been able to get itself invited to the policy-making tables (from which patients have been excluded) where it is decided how money is spent, which treatments merit support, and how research is coordinated for maximum efficiency. NBCC's articulate and capable leadership has represented women with breast cancer admirably.

But because of the nature of politics, the NBCC has also contributed to the isolation of breast cancer from problems that affect all cancer. The same handful of representatives of the national organization are chosen over and over to sit on all the panels, boards, and committees, and they have guarded their access jealously.

The organization has chosen to concentrate on a very few issues in depth and has done it effectively. But it has overwhelmed the voice of grassroots organizations with broader—or simply different—issues about breast cancer.

The Power of the Purse

In a very real sense, money talks. It is hard to tell the public anything about an organization, a disease, or an issue without sufficient money to do it in a way that has an impact.

One of the facts of cancer advocacy is that the money to finance it flows, as it does in nearly every other respect, from drug companies. Patient groups turn to the industry just as research facilities do—because that's where the money is. A consequence is that drug companies in many ways manipulate and influence what reaches the public about cancer.

Cancer Frontline

As part of CAN ACT's goal of educating and empowering patients to make informed treatment decisions, we published *Cancer Frontline*, which reported on selected clinical trials *in plain English* (no medical jargon) so people could understand what the trial was about and who could qualify. It was the first such periodical for the public.

Patients' *only* access to clinical-trial information until then was through the CIS 800-telephone number, which dispenses highly technical material for patients to *take to their doctors for interpretation*.

The first issue of *Cancer Frontline*—5,000 copies mailed *free* to individuals, hospitals, social workers, and oncologists—was funded by pooled contributions from two drug companies whose lawyers asked us not to thank them by name in print. They did not want to be identified with an organization that questioned FDA's policies on cancer drugs.

The *Frontline* had a very encouraging response. It was clear that it was a novel way to get valuable information to a receptive public.

The second issue featured a dozen trials in different cancers of *one* important new drug. The drug's manufacturer underwrote the cost of publication, but again attorneys would accept only the most inconspicuous appreciation, and that reluctantly. This time, 9,000 copies were distributed. Requests for additional copies came in for *years* afterward.

Much heartened, we moved to set up a more permanent publication that would guarantee four issues of *Frontline* a year and ensure medical consultation (for accuracy). We were encouraged to submit a detailed proposal and budget by the largest company in the oncology field, which underwrites patient groups very substantially. We were turned down. Instead, they funded a teary exhibit memorializing women who had died of breast cancer—another victory of the "poor patient" over information and education, of death over life.

What does that tell a would-be activist (perhaps you) about what gets funded? It is that *appearances count more than substance*. Drug companies want their names associated with feel-good public relations. They are as risk-averse as the FDA itself, and they run from controversy, especially from strong positions.

Just look at the number of publications sponsored by different companies on the same few topics. It's part of why there is so much psychosocial support material—who would argue with it?

But read a brochure about treatment with a new drug. You'd think the new drug was strawberry jam. Tiptoeing around the hard, sad facts of cancer treatment, you'd learn that you *might* lose your hair or that you *might* experience some nausea or discomfort.

The truth is that patient materials are produced and distributed by people who are afraid of cancer. And that fear communicates itself in a way that gives us a distorted picture of themselves.

The Power of the Press

The media is an important intermediary between the cancer advocate and the public, but they have their own views about how cancer should be portrayed, their own agenda. And guess what? It's sentimental, the "poor patient" story.

When you read a story in a newspaper about cancer or watch a segment on TV, almost all of the time it will feature a patient who is hurt by a drug, by a doctor, or by the system. You'll *never* see a strong, tough patient fighting the system, fighting the FDA or the NCI (unless the underlying story is that it's too little, too late). You'll never see or hear a thoughtful discussion of the issues or ideas. That may be your agenda, but the press goes for the tear every time.

This approach has two serious effects:

1. It shows us a picture of ourselves that distorts and undermines our own understanding of ourselves and our capabilities. If all we see are *emotion-laden, romanticized* images of *melodramatic,*

pathetic, resigned victims, how can we guess that it could be different or that there are people with different ideas? (Just say those words over a few times. Do they fit you? Are you comfortable with that description?)

2. It blocks the other message, that we have strengths and determination to draw on and that we can be motivated to act in our own cause. "You know how it is," a young producer will say. "We have to touch people's hearts first." But they never get to the brains.

The Power of the Peers

The last thing you'd imagine—rivalry among cancer patient organizations—may be the biggest obstacle to the development of effective cancer advocacy. Sadly, many organizations seem to lose sight of the larger issues in their drive to protect their financial, territorial, and publicity interests, tending the growth of the organization over the issues and interests of people with cancer.

The formation of subcoalitions or cliques in cancer organizations enlarges the turf and further defends them against newcomers that are more activist or more outspoken. People who sit on boards of each other's organizations collude in a way that would not be permitted in commerce.

Some cancer-patient organizations are very big businesses. The issues can wait while they assure their financing. Executives of voluntary health organizations are not volunteers; most make very respectable salaries.

Although stable funding is important, one must question the cost of such stability. The more funding derives from corporate sources, the more conservative and less activist an organization becomes because corporate sponsors don't want to offend.

The sad fact is that there are more than enough issues to go around, and more than enough funding. A great deal of talent is being wasted in cancer organizations, and the price of that is too high for everyone.

The Power of the Professional

We patients rarely get to speak for ourselves. The professionals speak for us in the media and in setting policies that affect us in institutions.

Every hospital's Institutional Review Board, for example, must approve clinical trials involving their patients. Because they are required to have consumer representation and because the vast majority of clinical trials involve cancer patients, you might think that informed cancer patients would frequently (or even occasionally) be found as members of IRB boards. In fact, the opposite is true. A random sampling of IRBs of large metropolitan hospitals turned up *no* consumer members who were other than medical or psychological practitioners—doctors, nurses, social workers, clergy, or professional "ethicists."

When there is a new development in cancer, the press quotes doctors, stock analysts, drug company executives, and (from time to time) the ACS, although they always telephone *activists* to get *accurate background information.* The press perpetuates the authoritarian, paternalistic structure of cancer while, at the same time, restricting other, more realistic, images of cancer from getting out.

When doctors are asked their opinions about treatment, quality-of-life issues or anything else, they evidently never think of asking us patients what we think nor of asking us to answer instead of themselves. In this regard, it appears they believe it is still their right and responsibility to act as patients' surrogates.

Perhaps it's the one-way street problem. In more than five years of CAN ACT's existence, no professional medical organization invited our views—even shared ones—or asked us to sit as equals on a panel at a medical meeting discussing, for example, mutual concerns regarding off-label drug use or insurance problems. In many instances, however, they generously cooperated with us, appearing at *our* public meetings to answer patients' treatment questions.

THE PEOPLE'S AGENDA: WHEN YOU WANT TO GET INVOLVED

The practical problems facing a would-be cancer activist are daunting. If you are convinced that you should do something, don't look at the big picture but only at the part of it *where you might fit in* by reason of your interests and knowledge. If you are to develop an interest in a cancer issue that can sustain you over the long term, through periods of heartbreaking frustration and maybe anger or pain, you must find something *you really care about* to work on.

Often the loss of someone close to us is sufficiently motivating: The founder of the Susan G. Komen Breast Cancer Foundation lost her sister to the disease, and the founder of The Mautner Project lost a beloved friend to breast cancer. Or it may be that the desire to master your own disease is sufficiently compelling (and why shouldn't it be?). Most people involved with grassroots cancer organizations come to advocacy from their own experience with the disease.

The Long Island Breast Cancer Studies

Long Island, a finger of land pointing eastward from New York City's Manhattan island, is home to women with among the highest rates of breast cancer in the nation. In response to pressure from residents for an explanation, four studies were undertaken by the state health authorities, each one concluding that dietary fat consumption by an indolent, upper-class, ethnic population was the root cause.

Needless to say, this was a very unpopular conclusion. Many women called it a "smoke screen" instead of a thorough analysis, pointing out that Long Island has unique conditions that warrant more serious study: All power lines are exposed; most of the land was agricultural until the 1950s, heavily fertilized and sprayed; drinking water is drawn from underground aquifers; and the island itself lies amid waters of questionable quality near several states' undersea dumping grounds. Contrary to the state's assumption, the population is educated and at least as aware of the need to follow a healthy diet and exercise program as anywhere else in the United States.

Critics pointed out many flaws in the design of the studies, including that known "hot spots," clusters of breast and other cancers, were not identified and studied. But the state, having appeared to discharge its duty (and in so doing, blaming the victims) refused to study the problem further.

It was not until women on Long Island mobilized, taking matters into their own hands, that they were able to break through bureaucratic rigidity. At that time, a few breast cancer groups held a rally to draw attention to the problem. Volunteers were enlisted for a house-by-house survey of the incidence of breast cancer in large areas of each of the two counties that comprise the island. An elaborate map was drawn up that graphically demonstrated that clusters of breast cancer exist and that they relate to the location of former industrial or agricultural sites.

The now-swelling numbers of breast cancer activists marshalled the support of local politicians in their cause, which was to have one *thorough* environmental study. Ultimately, political action brought the Centers for Disease Control and Prevention into the picture to lead what is intended to be a model study of the conditions that may cause breast cancer. Most tellingly, the NCI was forced by the alliance of activists and politicians to break its longstanding closed-door policy and to include local activists on the study's scientific advisory committee.

Women on Long Island are aware, involved, and activated now. They know that this is their fight.

Emerging Issues

There are ways for you to get involved in the fight against cancer that go beyond work with organizations strictly devoted to cancer policies. Many groups advocate positions that affect cancer in one way or another without making it their primary agenda. You might find it satisfying to work on some of the more challenging social problems that we face.

Prevention issues.   The agricultural industry has been lobbying the FDA to withdraw the Delaney Clause, which restricts the amount of pesticide residue permitted in prepared foods to essentially the minimal measureable levels. The FDA agrees that its way of measuring is out of date technologically. They know that we are taking in more residues than we think and that, although tested singly, the residues have cumulative effects. The FDA would like to overhaul the Delaney Clause, but many people fear that industry will dictate looser regulation. The agricultural industry would like to do away with all regulation.

What do you think about food additives? Should the agricultural industry be trusted to determine how much pesticide *you* will consume? Many food additives are carcinogens. If you care about these issues, you could work to ensure the safety of the food supply and to prevent cancer at the same time.

Talc, as in talcum powder, has been suspected *for decades* to be a cause of ovarian and lung cancers. The talc industry has lobbied the FDA in ways that hold off regulation year after year. There is simply no individual or group pushing for definitive research and a determination of the role of talc, so people are still exposed to it. The FDA says, "We just don't know."

Other suspected causes of cancer that have been insufficiently investigated until pressure from cancer advocates forced some small show of professional concern are low-frequency electromagnetic fields (such as are found around heat-generating small electrical appliances like electric blankets), overhead electrical power lines, and organochlorines, including chlorine in drinking water.

Treatment issues.   Many people work for the preservation of the environment for its own sake. But do you know how many new drugs have been developed from plants found in exotic rain forests and stands of ancient plants? The potential for discovering still more is very good—reason enough to preserve and protect the rain forest and farther reaches of the planet.

Taxol, the most useful new chemotherapeutic agent of the last few years, comes from the bark of a scarce Pacific yew that grows in age-old forests of the Pacific Northwest, habitat of some endangered species of birds. Harvesting the raw material set off conflicts among environmental preservationists, logging interests, and medical advocates because issues were raised that are not easily resolved. Several organizations, among them the Rain Forest Alliance, recognize the need to develop new medications, but to do it in such a way that the environment is protected for itself and for what it might yield in the future. You might tie interests you have together in this issue, benefiting both the planet and cancer.

And of course, the FDA, a boundless source of controversy, has numerous issues in which you might develop an interest. You could, for instance, speak at meetings of FDA advisory committees to urge faster cancer-drug approvals during the time open to the public (usually 8 A.M., which hardly encourages participation). Or you might investigate why AIDS drugs alone have the highest priority for approval and how this plays out in numbers of drugs approved over time compared with cancer drugs.

The NCI itself has arrogantly turned its back on real patient involvement in *its* important decisions by appointing the same two or three "acceptable" members of the public to its panels. It offers an attractive target for an activist, someone who might become interested in the ivory tower attitudes held by our largest publicly funded research institution.

Quality of care issues. Because the health insurance industry is so powerful and so poorly regulated, it has managed to set practices with hardly a fear of challenge. Now, as serious quality-of-care problems are being recognized, that may be changing.

In several states, coalitions of VHAs have directed their efforts toward the regulatory authorities to ensure that people enrolled in the new types of plans are receiving the quality of service they expect. This is a particularly fertile area for lawyers who want to do pro bono work: The regulations are complex, and regulators and regulated have more in common with each other than with you or me (one of the problems).

HOW TO FIND OR FOUND AN ADVOCACY GROUP

Let's define some terms: There is a distinction between *advocates* and *activists*, but it's a matter of interpretation; people may call themselves either. *Advocates* are often affiliated with middle-of-the-road organizations or medical institutions, like social workers who advocate for their patients. (The designation for lawyers in many languages is "advocate" because they are intermediaries who speak *in place of* their clients.) *Activists* speak for themselves, usually in a more direct manner. They often represent a small grassroots organization that does not have a conservative board of directors to be placated.

Grassroots groups spring up among the people who are directly affected by some problem or who share a concern. Many important shifts in public policy in our lifetime have their origins in independent grassroots organizations: groups that questioned the reasons for our being at war in Vietnam, such as Women's Strike for Peace and others; Mothers Against Drunk Driving (MADD), which confronted a misguided tolerance for drunk driving; People for the Ethical Treatment of Animals (PETA) and others reminding us that we do not have the right to abuse animals with which we share our planet.

Finding a Group

You can find a group in much the same way you'd go about finding a support group when you know what you want to do and when you understand how involved you want to be. (See Chapter 8.)

Many support groups are interested in expanding into advocacy, but they might not know what to do or how to go about it. You can make a place for yourself by simply announcing your intention. You might be surprised at how open the field is: You can do whatever you're willing to give the time for, because most people are not willing to give any. They don't know that that's what it takes.

You may be willing to start a chapter of a national organization in your area. It's much easier than starting from scratch because plenty of professional help and advice will be available. You will have instant legitimacy, but somewhat less autonomy. Becoming a chapter of a national organization may incur a financial obligation to the headquarters. Be sure you understand the details thoroughly.

Founding a Group

Detailed instruction on founding an organization is beyond the scope of this book. Talk to other people who have experience in grassroots organizing. In many communities, there are public-interest groups that can offer professional advice to people founding a self-help group. Every situation is different, but lots of the problems are the same.

An activist organization is very much about the founder's enthusiasm, dedication, and belief in the rightness of what she or he is doing. Gathering a group of diverse people equally motivated to do something about an issue as complicated as cancer isn't easy, not nearly so easy as getting neighbors to work together for block improvement or on a local civic problem. If you understand generally how to go about it and note the following special tips and caveats about cancer groups, you can make it work.

Make sure people understand how they are affected if you want them to respond. A small group of people with something important in common can be a productive beginning. Narrow the appeal for participation as much as you can. If you are focusing on one form of cancer, you can define the medical specialists, the segment of the patient population, and others (drug or biotech companies, for instance) that may be willing to help you.

Start small. If you can identify a group of people that is underserved or under-recognized, you can build a constituency among them that can be expanded later. Most organizations have two tiers of members: the core founders who do the work and the people who contribute money or who are on the mailing list, but are not more active than that. It's important to have a group behind you: It gives you validity with elected representatives, who count noses. (You have to be able to answer the inevitable question, "How many people do you represent?") Religious groups, one or another minority, and ethnic or professional associations are all potential constituents that are too infrequently drawn into activism.

Assign responsibilities to people. Grassroots organizing is the *hardest* thing, and the problems are classic. Idealism runs out quickly in the tough work of organization. Try to keep people involved by breaking responsibilities down into tasks. Most people are willing to be envelope-stuffers—they'll give an hour or two a week, but they are not interested in taking responsibility for anything, let alone thinking up what to do and how to do it.

The rest of the people are probably already overcommitted. Don't count on them for more than moral support. Keep reaching out for new people.

Build a solid board of directors. Most grassroots organizations begin with a board composed only of the idealistic do-gooders who founded the organization. *It just doesn't work.* Have a more business-like approach, including a plan for the growth of the organization.

You must attract corporate people to the board, people with contacts, access to contributions, and, above all, know-how. Lawyers and accountants should be available pro bono (for the benefit of the public—no cost to you) to do required paperwork for the organization. If you can't get corporate people, think seriously about your involvement.

Have a Plan of Action

1. *Draw up a statement of purpose.* It will help you clarify the issues, explain the background, and make your case in a concise, clear way. Make a background study of the situation and what has been done to correct it, if anything. Explain why the situation is dangerous, inadequate, or otherwise important to change and what obstacles exist. Print it up in a flyer or a brochure.

2. *Make a funding plan.* It's hard to develop a realistic funding plan when you're starting out, but short-term plans are necessary. The board should have enough personal responsibility and involvement to fund the start-up costs. Learn to write grant proposals (it's not too difficult) and appeal to the companies that benefit from the cancer on which you are working. Ask for money for a specific project with which they would like to be associated. Almost no one will fund overhead, so you must squeeze it out of grants and contributions. Anyone with experience in funding will explain it, and there are books about fund-raising for nonprofits.

Tip: If you plan to seek funding from drug companies, be sure your plans include nice-nice projects. You can hope for funding for educational projects but not for activist or political efforts.

3. *Have a public event to attract more people.* When you have the nucleus of a group, plan a rally, a walk, or a meeting to recruit more people into your group. You need plenty of hands to manage the group and to do fund-raising, media contact, desktop publishing, and other tasks. Many people are less interested in the activist agenda than in information or in the benefit they want for themselves, but their presence will help you meet your own goals.

4. *Alert your target.* When the group has solidified, communicate with the target. Let them know you exist. State your concerns in a letter and ask for a meeting with the chief executive to discuss them. Then send out a press release, a mailing to your list, and a communication to other groups about your progress.

5. *Build coalitions.* This is useful but tricky because of petty interorganizational jealousies. You might need each other's support, so forge careful alliances with groups whose views are compatible with yours. Not every cancer group is on the same side of the fence, nor can they agree on everything, so proceed slowly in this.

6. *Get politicians behind you.* Local representatives will be glad to hear they have another constituency to represent. Make yourselves

known, perhaps by inviting a representative and aides to a public meeting. They can connect you with related groups or with possible sources of funding. If your district or federal representatives sit on committees that affect what you do, so much the better. Otherwise, ask for introductions.

7. *Choose your tactics.* Whatever you are going to do, do it so you maximize the return. If you can accomplish a goal and build public support at the same time, it's more efficient. It's certainly better to bring the public along with you than to antagonize it by obstructionist tactics.

8. *Include the media.* Although it's problematic, the media decides what makes news, so it must be taken into consideration. If you plan a public event, do something *visual.* The more attention-getting the event, the more likely you are to get someone out to cover it. When you are in the press, it puts you on the map. Have someone learn to write good press releases. Fax them out frequently, and have them prepared as handouts. It's the way news happens.

Tip: If you work with the media, *always make "human interest" your opening.* Start a story with the patient angle, have a patient ready to go on camera or to tell a story. You can always make the important point later. But first you've got to get the media's attention.

Working Alone

For perfectly sensible reasons, you may not want to find *or* found a group. There are things you can do alone that will give you a sense of satisfaction and contribute to the overall progress of cancer, but not take the time or intense involvement that other kinds of undertakings would.

Julie (see Chapter 4) did not have time or energy to devote to an advocacy group, even if there were one in the almost-rural area in which she lives. But her dynamic nature, and her awareness of what shrinking budgets will mean for cancer research at NIH, helped her decide to do what she could. You'll find her now at public meetings and political gatherings, always with a sheaf of petitions supporting sustained levels of research funding.

She's become a fixture at her Senate and Congressional offices, where she also volunteers some time. Her elected representatives, local and federal, know her well. She helps them understand her perspective on cancer issues, and she follows closely how they vote on them. Local newspapers seek her informed opinions when health issues arise, so she is helping to educate the public. She is one person who is making a difference all by herself and feeling good about it.

Burnout

A discussion of grassroots activism would be incomplete without mentioning the possibility (or probability) of burnout. Suitably warned against doing too much yourself, you are probably going to end up doing just that. Other people will tell you that they'd love to help, but they're too busy, or they have to get back to work, or they'll call when they're feeling better. But keep up the good work, they urge.

If you're spending a lot of time frustrated or feeling spread too thin or angry, recognize these little flares as warning of burnout ahead. When you're feeling the heat, step back and evaluate what can be done in the time you *want* to spend doing it, or consider stepping back altogether.

An entire generation of activists (but not the "advocates") has burnt out in the past five years, their dedication, drive, and energy consumed by the movement. It's something to think about.

There is a tide in the events of men (and women). Not every movement, every group, *should* go on indefinitely. There is something useful and healthy about doing what you can and moving on, especially if you can feel you've made a difference. The more general and mainstream the ideas are that you espouse, the more likely they are to find wide acceptance. That kind of advocacy doesn't usually erode the psyche, although it may keep you very busy. Trying to do more, to do it faster—that's what leads to frustration.

MOVING ON

Four years after CAN ACT was founded, I had a heart-to-heart talk late one evening with a cancer journalist who had covered the development of cancer patient advocacy from its beginning. We were sitting in the almost-deserted bar of a midwestern airport hotel at the end of a two-day conference. I understood, after four years, what it *really* meant to try to have an impact on government policies, the near impossibility of it, and I was depressed.

As I spoke to him of my frustration, tears came to my eyes. I was too drained to care. My friend, though, was surprised. He enumerated all that I and CAN ACT had accomplished, reminding me that no other patient organization had dared challenge the FDA on issues so critical to treatment.

"I've been doing this for four years. What real change have we got to show for it?" I asked.

"You don't understand," he replied. "Four years is the blink of an eye to the government. But look what you did: You got it to blink."

CAN ACT forced the cancer community to recognize and confront crucial issues of access to treatment that affect people with every type of cancer. As the first cancer activists, we influenced the agenda of other organizations, which in many instances enlarged from psychosocial support to advocacy.

That development has allowed me to move in a different direction: out of the line of fire. No more patronizing from bureaucrats for me; no more condescension from people who care more for power than principle. Now I contemplate thinking and writing about cancer issues in tranquility.

In 1995, the oft-cited pendulum has suddenly swung, as it will, too far in the other direction. I'm shocked to find myself defending the need for an FDA to critics who would *completely* dismantle the agency. Are we ready for a return to "caveat emptor"? It's not what I had in mind. I'll sit this one out.

Ten years ago, I bargained with the Fates to live long enough to see my child grow into adulthood. I trust they will consider my debt paid in dedication.

RECOMMENDED READING

Following are the titles of an eclectic collection of publications I've found informative, helpful, or inspiring. There are many medically oriented books about specific cancers and their treatment, but they are not on this list. These are about empowerment.

And the Band Played On: Politics, People and the AIDS Epidemic, by Randy Shilts (New York: St. Martin's Press, 1987).

The indisputable classic. Powerfully written, it walks you through the development of AIDS activism so you understand more about the way things really were. And still are.

Against the Odds: The Story of AIDS Drug Development, Politics & Profits, by Peter Arno and Karyn Feiden (New York: HarperCollins, 1992).

Another view from the AIDS community. This book focuses on the corporate politics and economics of drug development in the context of public policy in healthcare.

Grass Roots: How Ordinary People Are Changing America, by Tom Adams (New York: Citadel Press, 1991).

How grassroots organizations such as Act Up, Mothers Against Drunk Driving (MADD), and People for the Ethical Treatment of Animals (PETA) got started in response to common concerns or grievances. Adams explains how groups differ in their structure, tactics, and outreach. A revealing selection of press releases and letters concluding the book shows the cynical manipulation of a citizens' animal-rights group by a large corporation that professed to be changing its policies on animal testing.

"I Love You, Too!", by Woodrow Wirsig (New York: M. Evans & Co., 1990).

Woody's moving story of his wife, Jane, as Alzheimer's disease stole her life. After trying a range of alternative and untested therapies, he learned of THA, which reversed her illness for two precious years. He had to fight the FDA every inch of the way for the unapproved drug, which was only approved years later as Cognex, the first drug to show any effect against Alzheimer's. The book tells more of their personal story than politics, but it documents the same federal mindset toward patient advocacy as exists for cancer.

The Dread Disease: Cancer and Modern American Culture, by James T. Patterson (Cambridge: Harvard University Press, 1987).

The fascinating cultural history of cancer in our time. Patterson, a political historian, provides indispensible background for understanding how the issues of cancer affected the views of professionals, government, and the populace. That the periodic emergence of cancer activists is needed to renew the commitment to curing cancer is depressing, given the statistics, except that better treatment is the result for many kinds of cancer.

Oncology Times (New York: J. B. Lippincott Co).

A monthly, large-format, news magazine written for oncology professionals in a clear, popular style that is accessible to the knowledgeable lay reader. At this time, a yearly subscription is $90 (For information, call 800-638-3030; in Maryland, call 301-714-2300 collect.)

Trauma and Recovery, by Judith Herman, M.D. (New York: Basic Books, 1992).

Dr. Herman, an Associate Clinical Professor of Psychiatry at the Harvard Medical School, has written extensively about the process of recovery from public or private traumatic experience. In this book, she shows how victims of different kinds of violence, such as childhood abuse, sexual mistreatment of women, and men's experiences in war, share fundamental psychological similarities. You may not agree, but I find many parallels with cancer. Her perspectives on recovery, on empowerment, and on reintegration of the self after a powerful threat (such as that posed by cancer), are not easy reading but are very convincing.

Searching for Magic Bullets: Orphan Drugs, Consumer Activism, and Pharmaceutical Development, by Lisa Basara and Michael Montagne (New York: Pharmaceutical Products Press, 1994).

A thorough as well as entertaining survey of the American pharmaceutical industry that will help you understand the tangle of economic, ethical and regulatory issues that prolong the process of drug development and approval. Special attention is paid to orphan drugs. Although it is written from a strongly consumer-protectionist point of view, this little book is full of information for anyone interested in making a serious study of the topic.

The FDA Follies, An Alarming Look at Our Food and Drugs in the 1980s, by Herbert Burkholz (New York: Basic Books, 1994).

A contrarian view: The FDA is the hero! Interesting reading, especially as we may be entering another era of deregulation.

Outrageous Practices: The Alarming Truth about How Medicine Mistreats Women, by Leslie Laurence and Beth Weinhouse (New York: Fawcett Columbine, 1994).

If women only read the chapter "Women and Doctors," this book will be galvanizing enough. The rest of it should thoroughly convince you of the need to become an empowered, educated medical consumer *before* you find yourself in a medical crisis.

Patenting the Sun: Polio and the Salk Vaccine, by Jane Smith (New York: William Morrow & Co., 1990).

The last dread disease of our era before AIDS. Once again, big science and big personalities in an era of big government. It's interesting to consider the social context, remembering how and why FDR concealed his polio from the public and especially from photographers.

Choices in Healing/Integrating the Best of Conventional and Complementary Approaches to Cancer, by Michael Lerner (Cambridge, MA: The MIT Press, 1994).

Lerner believes in an integrated approach to treating cancer but argues that information from any discipline is hard to come by. His valuable contribution is to identify what is known—and not kown—about the usefulness of treatment practices from mainstream medicine through unconventional pharmacological, psychological, and traditional ones.

INDEX

ABOUT THE AUTHOR

Beverly Zakarian is executive director and cofounder of CAN ACT, the first activist cancer-patient organization and the first to identify the critical role of the FDA in the survival of people with the disease. As the spokesperson for a unique organization, Ms. Zakarian has represented patient views before Congress, the President's Cancer Panel, and the FDA. She has written numerous articles about treatment issues. Prior to being diagnosed with ovarian cancer in 1985, she was a graphic designer and writer, coauthor of *College Appli-kit*, a self-help application guide for high school students.